The Eas
Air Fryer Cookbook

Full-Coloured Book with Quick and Delicious Recipes for Every Occasion

Nancy Bailey

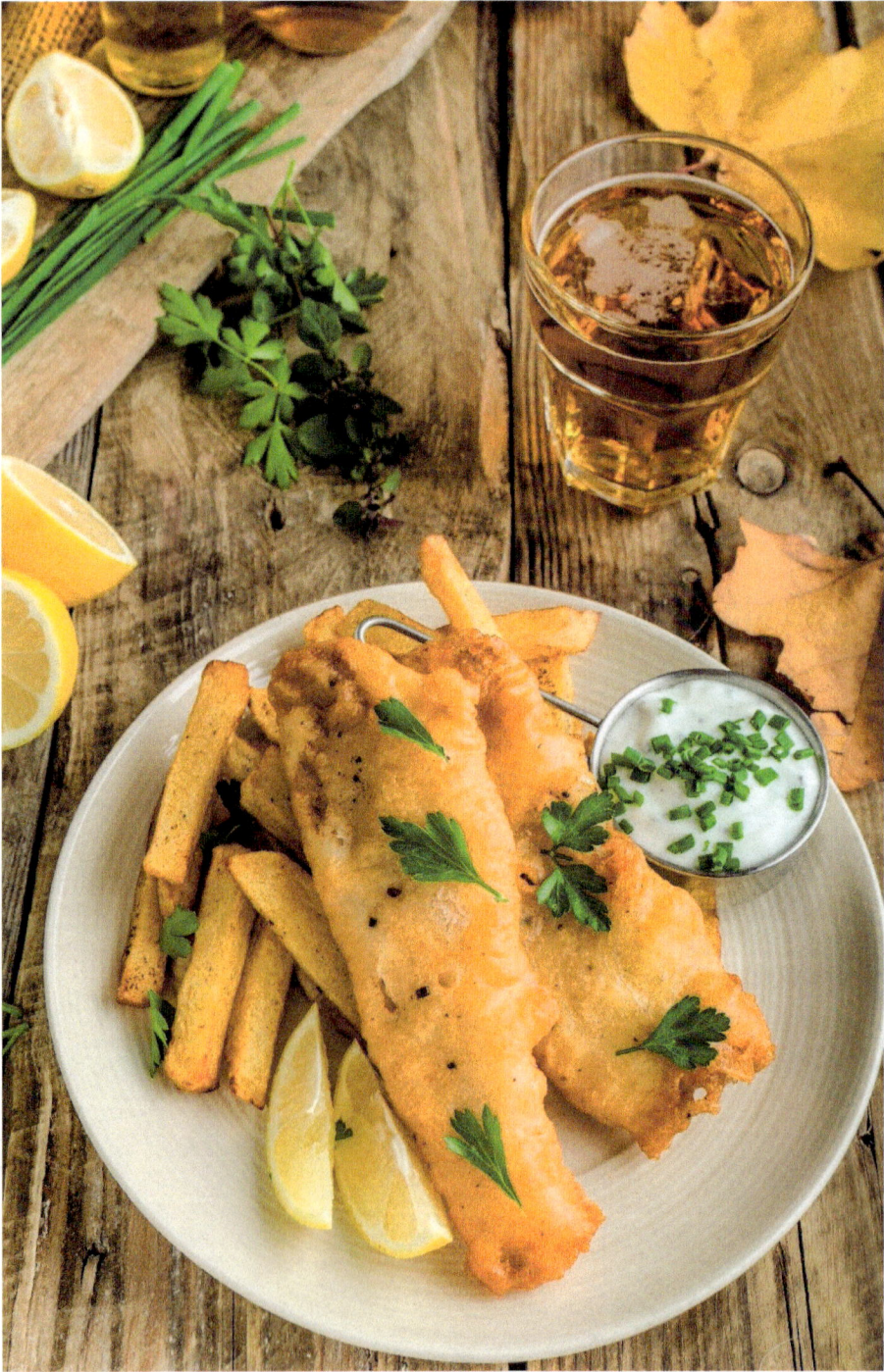

TABLE OF CONTENTS

INTRODUCTION

Air Fryers have started to become popular, due to the fact that you can avoid many of the unhealthy aspects of modern cooking. But what is an Air Fryer exactly, and how on earth does it work?

Air Fryers are basically an upgraded, enhanced countertop oven, but they became popular for one particular reason. In fact, many of the manufacturers, such as Philips, market this machine solely based on the claim that the Air Fryers accurately mimic deep-frying, which, although extremely unhealthy, is still very popular in this day and age (as it is, in my opinion, one of the most delicious ways to eat food).

Air Fryers work with the use of a fan and a heating mechanism. You place the food you want cooked in a basket or on the rack, turn on the machine, and the Air Fryer distributes oven-temperature hot air around your food. It provides consistent, pervasive heat evenly to all the food within. This heat circulation achieves the crispy taste and texture that is so tantalizing in deep fried foods, but without the unhealthy and dangerous oil! Both have been replaced by this miracle machine with hot air and a fan.

ADVANTAGES TO USING AN AIR FRYER

I may have already slipped in a few of the advantages to using an Air Fryer, but now let's expand a little more on everything an Air Fryer can do for you. After all, no investment should be made unless it's absolutely worthwhile.

And in truth, the Air Fryer is very worthwhile. I cannot begin to tell you how the advantages start piling up; this is not just another average appliance that everyone is getting because of a simple trend. People are getting Air Fryers because of their incredible, numerous, multifaceted benefits.

There are, however, a few notable advantages of using an Air Fryer, which I'll list below. If you don't know anything else about Air Fryers, I hope that these will convince you of their worth.

HEALTHIER COOKING

This is perhaps the top benefit that comes with air frying. In a society that really struggles with healthy cooking, we can use all the help we can get. Luckily, Air Fryers make it easy, all while maintaining many of the factors that make unhealthy food delicious!
Air Fryers use very little oil, which is one of the best ways to replace those unhealthy fried foods, like fried chicken, potatoes, and so many others. If you are like me (a lover of deep fried foods) then this is the answer to your dilemma of healthy eating while still enjoying the crispy taste of food!

Do keep in mind that you still need to spray fried foods, such as fish, with a touch of oil to make sure it does get evenly crispy. All in all, however, there is no denying the amount of oils is a whole lot less.

This singular change makes all the difference in the world. Healthy eating has never been easier, as you'll get the same crispy and flavorsome results, with minimal amounts of added oils. You'll even be able to "fry" foods you never were able to before—the possibilities are endless!

SAFER AND EASIER

Nothing scares me more than a hot pot of oil. It is an accident waiting to happen, and getting struck with burning oil splatters is no joke! But this, and its corresponding injuries, is often the price to pay for deep fried foods.

Air Fryers are also user-friendly, and this makes a huge difference. You don't have to feel like you are studying for a degree when working with an Air Fryer. Making dinner is far less complicated in an Air Fryer than many of the traditional methods of cooking. For some meals—unless you choose one of the more complex recipes I'll share later—you can even revert to placing a small piece of meat (even if it happens to be frozen!) into the basket and select the cooking settings.

The simplicity of the Air Fryer is its beauty. You will save countless time and unnecessary frustrations, and still make delicious food!

FASTER THAN COOKING IN THE OVEN

Once you buy an Air Fryer and set it to heat for the first time, you won't know what hit you! The average normal oven needs about 10 minutes to preheat. Due to the Air Fryer's smaller size and innovative design, it will be ready to go in no time!

It's even faster during the actual cooking. With the circulation that allows your food to be cooked crisp and even, it cuts a whole lot of cooking time out of the equation. This is amazing, especially in this day and age where technology, work, friends, family, and even pets are constantly demanding our attention.

Just imagine! You could set your food in the Air Fryer, and (with some recipes) it will be ready to eat in less than 20 minutes!

SAVES SPACE

If you are someone living in a small apartment, or a student accommodation, then an Air Fryer is perfect for you. Air Fryers are much smaller in comparison to a conventional oven and you can easily make use of this Air Fryer in 1 cubic foot of your kitchen.

You can even pack your Air Fryer away after use if need be, but the majority of people choose to keep it out on the counter. But it's nice to have the option to move your Air Fryer around if space becomes an issue.

LOW OPERATING COSTS

Considering how much cooking oil costs these days and the amount you need to use, you will soon be cutting costs in making deep fried foods. All an Air Fryer uses is a small amount of oil and some of the electricity to power up the Air Fryer, about the same amount that a countertop oven would.

Not only will you be cutting out the massive oil costs, which will save money, you will likely also save money by ordering out less, as you'll be able to replicate your favorite foods quickly and easily at home!

NO OIL SMELL

In reality, smelling like the food you just ate is not impressive, regardless of how delicious the food may be. This is what often happens, however, when people enjoy deep fried foods.

When deep frying foods, it also causes the whole house to smell, and as the oil splatters around, it can leave a massive mess. The oil can even harden on the walls, causing grime to build up into a nasty concentration of dirt and grease.

With less cooking oil, Air Fryers don't have any of those oil smells and keeps the space cleaner around you, as all the oils, smells, and actual cooking are contained within the machine.

PRESERVES NUTRIENTS

When you are cooking your food in an Air Fryer, it actually protects a lot of the food from losing all its moisture. This means that with the use of a little oil, as well as circulation with hot air, it can allow your food to keep most of its nutrients which is excellent for you!

If you want to cook healthy foods with the purpose of maintaining as many nutrients as possible, then an Air Fryer is perfect for you!

EASIER TO CLEAN

Cleaning is perhaps the bane of my existence, especially after cooking and having a long day. This can really take away a lot of the pleasure of making yourself a great meal. But an Air Fryer lightens the burden by being easy to clean!

Consistent cleaning after using it (much like any pot or pan) can allow for easier and simpler living. You just need some soapy water and a non-scratch sponge to clean both the exterior and the interior of your Air Fryer. Some Air Fryers are even dishwasher-safe!

GREAT FLAVOUR

The flavour of Air Fryer "fried" foods is nearly identical to traditional frying, and the texture is exact. You can cook a lot of those great frozen foods, such as onion rings or french fries, and still achieve that crunchy effect. This certainly can help you turn to healthier foods, especially if your goal is for healthy but quality meals.

The Air Fryer helps to cook your food to perfect crispness, instead of the soggy mess that happens when you try alternative methods of cooking foods that are meant to be deep fried (like chicken tenders). No one really enjoys mushy food. The Air Fryer keeps that desired element while remaining healthy.

All you will really need is just some cooking oil sprayed outside of your food to end up with a cooked interior and a crunchy exterior. So no worries! You still can eat your foods with a crunch and a healthier result!

VERSATILE

Unlike rice cookers meant just for rice, or bread makers meant just for bread, you will find that an Air Fryer leaves a lot of room to be both versatile and healthier. You can cook almost anything you would like in the Air Fryer (as long as it fits). From spaghetti squash, to desserts, even to fried chicken! You will probably never run out of air frying options!

VARIOUS TYPES OF AIR FRYERS AND HOW TO CHOOSE THE ONE FOR YOU

There isn't one standardized choice of Air Fryers, which means you are far more likely to find an Air Fryer that really suits your particular needs. Whether it be size or price, you have a wider variety of choices than what normally comes with conventional ovens.

So what are the key aspects that you need to take into consideration when getting yourself a nice Air Fryer? Let's begin:

- **Dimensions:** Obviously they come in different sizes, and despite saving space, some can still be bulky. When thinking about your countertop, you do want to consider its size and dimensions. You don't want to play a game of tilt with your Air Fryer, nor have it taken up all the extra space you have!

- **Safety Features:** You may want to check that it has an auto shutoff, as it is certainly a desirable feature. Air Fryers can get very hot during use, and an auto-shutoff can save you a lot of stress and fire emergencies. Furthermore, having a cool exterior can prevent potential red and burnt hands. So do yourself a favour and make sure they have all these elements at hand.

- **Reviews:** Naturally, this is the best thing to check out. Considering that the businesses rarely give out all the information, you will certainly find it out when people leave reviews. The customer hides nothing, and if they are unhappy, they make sure everyone else knows about it. However, if people are very happy, many of them will also note it in the reviews, and it is best to target the Air Fryers that tend to have the high reviews.

TWO COMMON DIFFERENCES

Beyond those functional differences, there are two mainstream designs of Air Fryers: basket Air Fryers and oven Air Fryers. Each has very unique and distinguished features in which to enjoy. Let us take a look at the differences between the two:

BASKET AIR FRYERS

Basket fryers are known to need less space than oven Air Fryers, which is very practical if you have limited space. Not only does it save space, but it also saves time, as the food is quickly heated up (without unnecessarily heating up the kitchen). Unlike an oven Air Fryer, and the larger traditional oven, it only takes about 1-2 minutes for the basket Air Fryer to heat up, and it is quite easy to place the foods inside of the basket.

The cons are, for one, that it does make a lot more noise than the oven Air Fryer. You also will not be able to watch the food as it cooks, which can increase the chances of burnt food if you are not careful. Also, a basket Air Fryer may not be the best if you need to cook a lot of food, as it is limited in capacity. This means that batch cooking may be required if you need a large amount of food.

This makes a basket Air Fryer ideal if you have a limited budget, don't need to cook a huge amount of food, and have limited free time. They are quick, small, and convenient, especially perfect for people who are students or single working professionals, and maybe even you!

OVEN AIR FRYERS

Oven Air Fryers, in contrast, have a larger capacity, which means you can cook a lot more food at the same time. They also have multiple functions for cooking and cut down on the noise than the basket Air Fryer. You will also be able to move the food closer or even further away from the heating element. There is a lot more flexibility involved in the use of an oven Air Fryer. Best of all, you can place parts of the oven Air Fryer into the dishwasher to be washed (thus cutting down the cleaning process, if you happen to have a dishwasher).

But, do be aware that it takes up more counter space, and takes a larger initial bite out of your wallet. It may also heat up the kitchen more, and if you are in fashion and aesthetic design, it might be disappointing to find out the colours and themes are more limited than basket Air Fryers.

These are the two main common types of Air Fryers; however, there are new types of Air Fryers that are coming to light for you to use and enjoy, most notably, the paddle-type Air Fryer. This version has a paddle that moves through the basket of your Air Fryer in order to help circulate hot air in between each piece of food.

This saves you the effort of pulling your food out at a specific time and shaking or stirring it. These can also be noisy, and heat up the space, and are not small and convenient; however, if you are someone looking for convenience, then this is the Air Fryer to go for.

ACCESSORY TOOLS FOR AIR FRYER COOKING

I love how Air Fryers save time, so I've compiled a list of my favourite time-saving tools that I often use when meal prepping with my Air Fryer. Anything to help make your life easier and healthier should certainly be considered, and what better way to help than by adding some accessories to your Air Fryer inventory?

MANDOLINE

Preparation is always needed before jumping into air frying, and getting yourself the mandoline slicer is the perfect tool to slice online rings, pickles, or even the best and crunchiest chips. You can select the thickness or thinness, depending on what the recipe needs and says, so you will always be able to get the perfect crispness.

GRILL PAN

This is simply a pan created with a perforated surface. With this tool, you can both grill and sear foods like fish or even vegetables inside your Air Fryer. They are also commonly non-stick, which really helps your overall cleanup.

However, before you purchase a grill pan, make sure the Air Fryer model you have does support the grill pan. The last thing you want is to find that your grill pan just does not fit inside your Air Fryer.

HEAT RESISTANT TONGS

There is no denying how hot an Air Fryer can get inside, and unless you are a superhero, you will need some help manoeuvring in foods in and outside of the basket if need be. Using heat-resistant tongs can really make your life infinitely easier by keeping your foods, and your hands, safe. They are affordable, and really useful to allow for an even cooking process.

AIR FRYER LINERS

If you'd like to further decrease your clean-up time, then this is for you! These liners are both non-stick and non-toxic, making this a classic little investment for you to consider. They prevent the food from sticking to your Air Fryer and help in the process of keeping your little machine clean. You will not have to worry about burnt foods inside your fryer again!

AIR FRYER RACK

This adds a little bit more versatility as you can really take advantage of the surface cooking. With a rack, you ensure that heat is evenly distributed to all 360 degrees of your food. They are very safe and easy to use, and they increase the number of dishes you can cook at the same time

BAKING PANS

With an Air Fryer, you can even bake! You just need the right equipment, such as a barrel or round pan. With this you can even bake pizza, bread, muffins, and more. Imagine telling people you baked your own cake with an Air Fryer!

SILICONE BAKING CUPS

From egg bites to muffins, these are individual cups you can use in order to help compensate for the smaller space within an Air Fryer. The silicone material is heat-resistant, and allows for easier release of the contents, which spares you a lot of time cleaning. If you are a fan of baking, then this is a must have.

OIL SPRAYER

Naturally, one of the top benefits is needing much less oil when cooking with an Air Fryer, but it does not necessarily mean that you can cook with no oil at all. An oil sprayer is the key to getting the food you want to that nice golden-brown. You can use any oil that you like to use when cooking; all you need is a little spritz before you close the machine, and you are set!

THERMAPEN

Having the right cooking time is very important, but temperature also counts for a lot, and this is a nice little accessory to add to your collection. Having an instant-read thermometer can ensure all the food you have is cooked (and evenly so). If you are not completely certain at what temperatures food should be, you can always check out the various different guides.

HOW TO CLEAN AN AIR FRYER

As mentioned before, an Air Fryer is really easy to clean, but that doesn't mean you'll never need to clean it! Also, please remember that the cleanliness of your machine depends on how often you use it, and what you use it for.

It is recommended that you clean your Air Fryer after every use. As tempting as it may be to skip a day, it really is not worth it over the long run.

And that is the first step that comes with cleaning an Air Fryer:

- Do not delay the cleaning. Simply don't. Allowing crumbs or random bits of food to harden overnight can turn an easy task into a nightmare of a chore. If you do happen to air-fry foods that come with a form of sticky sauce, then the warmer they are, the easier again they will be to clean and remove.

- Unplug the machine, and use warm and soapy water to properly remove the dirt and components. You do not want anything abrasive in there. If there is food that gets stuck, try soaking it until it is soft enough to remove.

- If there is any food that happens to be stuck on the grate or in the basket, then you should consider gently using a toothpick or even a wooden skewer to scrape it off, in order to be thorough with your cleaning process.

- Remember to wipe the inside with a damp, soapy cloth, and remember to remove both the drawer and the basket.

- Finally, wipe the outside of your Air Fryer with a damp cloth or a sponge.

If there are any odors that seem to be stuck to your Air Fryer after cooking a strong food, even after you have cleaned it, then you can consider using a product called NewAir.

Just soak it in with water for about 3o minutes to an hour before you clean it. If the smell remains, then rub one lemon half over the drawer and the basket. Allow it to soak for another 30 minutes before washing it again.

Please do be careful with any non-stick appliances. They are a wonder for cleaning, but they can flake or come off over time. Be gentle, as you do not want anything to scratch or to even chip the coating. Not only does it ruin a little bit of the aesthetic look, a small part of your Air Fryer will constantly be struggling with sticky food.

There you have it! The first stepping stones and foundational knowledge of an Air Fryer. The device you will choose, and how you will use it is up to you, but there are still so many exciting varieties, choices, and options to come!

BANANA MUFFINS

10 minutes

20 minutes

18

INGREDIENTS

- 2 ripe bananas
- 150g self-raising flour
- 60g brown sugar
- 1 egg
- 60ml olive oil
- 60ml buttermilk
- Maple syrup, to brush, plus extra (optional), to serve

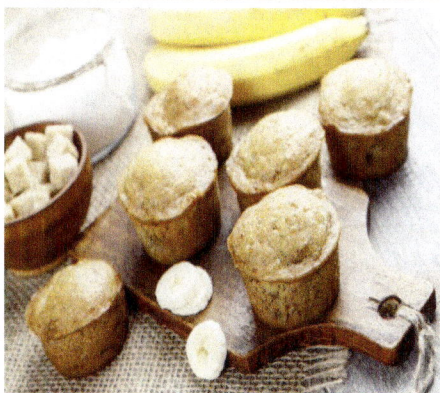

DIRECTIONS

1. Use a fork to mash the bananas in a small bowl and set aside.
2. Using a balloon whisk, beat the flour and sugar in a medium bowl. Form a hole in the centre and pour in the egg, oil and buttermilk. Use the whisk to break up the egg then with a wooden spoon, stir until the mixture is combined. While stirring, add the banana and mix everything together.
3. Preheat an air fryer to 180C. Divide half of the mixture among 9 patty cases. Remove the rack from the air fryer and transfer the cases to the rack then cook for 8-10 minutes. Transfer to a wire rack. Repeat with the remaining mixture to make 18 muffins.
4. Brush the tops of the muffins with maple syrup while still warm. Serve with extra maple syrup, if you like.

Nutrition: Calories: 105; Fat: 4 g; Protein: 2.5 g; Carbs: 15 g; Fibre: 0.5 g; Sugar: 7 g

CINNAMON ROLLS

15 minutes   10 minutes   6

INGREDIENTS

For The Rolls

- 2 tbsp. melted butter, plus more for brushing
- 75 g packed brown sugar
- 1/2 tsp. ground cinnamon
- Salt
- Plain flour, for surface
- 225 g ready rolled pizza dough

For The Glaze

- 50 g cream cheese, softened
- 65 g icing sugar
- 1 tbsp. whole milk, plus more if needed

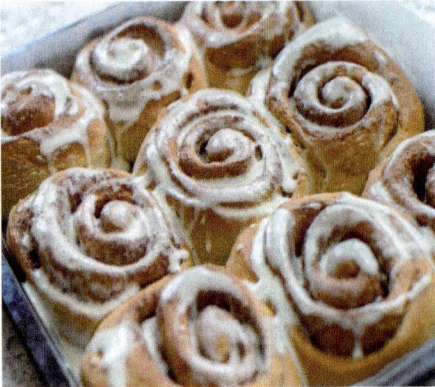

DIRECTIONS

1. Prepare the rolls: Line the bottom of the fryer with parchment paper and brush with butter. In a medium bowl, mix together the butter, brown sugar, cinnamon, and a large pinch of salt until smooth and fluffy.
2. On a lightly floured surface, roll out the dough into one piece. Pinch the seams and fold them in half. Roll out to a 22cm x 18cm rectangle.
3. Spread the butter mixture over the dough, leaving a 1.5cm border. Roll up the dough starting on the long side, then cut crosswise into 6 pieces.
4. Place the pieces, cut-side up, evenly spaced in the air fryer basket.
5. Set the fryer to 180°C and air fry for about 10 minutes, until they are golden brown and cooked through.
6. Prepare the frosting: In a medium bowl, beat together the cream cheese, powdered sugar, and milk. If needed, add more milk using a teaspoon to thin the glaze.
7. Spread the glaze on warm cinnamon rolls and serve.

Nutrition: Calories: 251; Fat: 8 g; Protein: 3 g; Carbs: 39 g; Fibre: 0.5 g; Sugar: 22

BACON MUFFINS

7 minutes

6 minutes

1

INGREDIENTS

- 1 Large Egg
- 1 Slice of Unsmoked Bacon
- 1 English All Butter Muffin
- 2 Slices of Burger Cheese
- 1 Pinch of Salt and Pepper

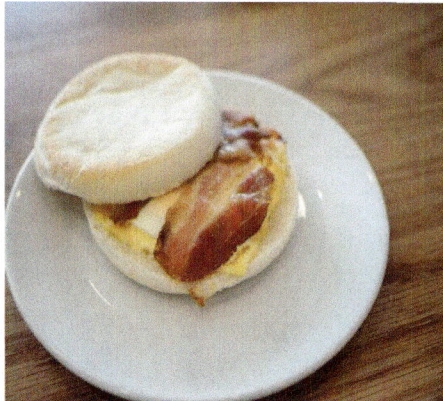

DIRECTIONS

1. Crack the large egg into either a ramekin or oven proof dish
2. Slice the muffin in half
3. Layer 1 slice of burger cheese on 1 half
4. Place now the muffin and bacon in the Air Fryer drawer, place the ovenproof dish or ramekin in the drawer too.
5. Heat up the Air Fryer to 200°C for 6 minutes
6. Once is done, assemble the breakfast muffin and add the extra slice of cheese on top.

Nutrition: Calories: 291; Fat: 12 g; Protein: 15 g; Carbs: 25 g; Fibre: 2 g; Sugar: 0 g

CHOCOLATE CHIP COOKIES

10 minutes

15 minutes

12

INGREDIENTS

- 115 g butter, melted
- 55 g brown sugar
- 50 g caster sugar
- 1 large egg
- 1 tsp. pure vanilla extract
- 185 g plain flour
- 1/2 tsp. bicarbonate of soda
- 1/2 tsp. salt
- 120 g chocolate chips
- 35 g chopped walnuts

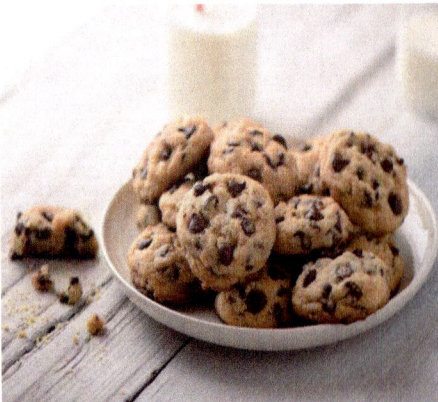

DIRECTIONS

1. Take medium bowl and whisk together melted butter and sugars.
2. Add egg and vanilla, whisk until incorporated.
3. Add salt, flour, bicarbonate of soda and stir.
4. Arrange a small piece of parchment in the Air Fryer's basket, making sure there is air flow around the edges.
5. Work in batches, using a large cookie scoop and scoop dough onto parchment, about 3 tablespoons, leaving 5cm between each of them, press to flatten slightly.
6. Bake in the Air Fryer at 180°C for 8 minutes. Cookies will be golden and slightly soft. Let them cool 5 minutes before serving.

Nutrition: Calories: 224; Fat: 13 g; Protein: 3.5 g; Carbs: 24 g; Fibre: 2 g; Sugar: 12 g

BACON-AND-EGGS AVOCADO

5 minutes

17 minutes

1

INGREDIENTS

- 1 large egg
- 1 avocado, halved, peeled, and pitted
- slices bacon
- Fresh parsley, for serving (optional)
- Sea salt flakes, for garnish (optional)

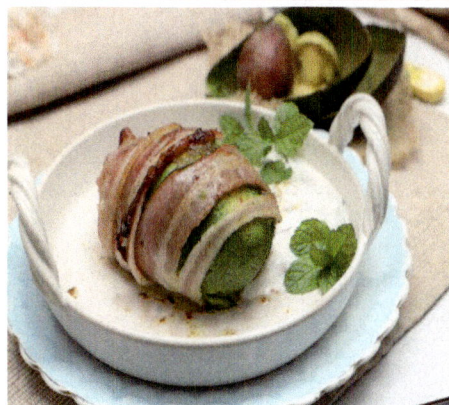

DIRECTIONS

1. Set the air fryer basket with avocado oil. Preheat the air fryer to 160 C. Fill a small bowl with cool water.
2. Soft-boil the egg: Place the egg in the air fryer basket. Air fry for 6 min for a soft yolk or 7 min for a cooked yolk. Bring the egg to the bowl of cool water and let sit for 2 min. Peel and set aside.
3. Use a spoon to carve out extra space in the centre of the avocado halves until the cavities are big enough to fit the soft-boiled egg. Place the soft-boiled egg in the centre of one half of the avocado and replace the other half of the avocado on top, so the avocado appears whole on the outside.
4. Starting at one end of the avocado, wrap the bacon around the avocado to completely cover it.
5. Place the bacon-wrapped avocado in the air fryer basket and air fry for 5 min. Flip the avocado over and air fry for another 5 min or until the bacon is cooked to your liking. Serve on a bed of fresh parsley, if desired, and sprinkle with salt flakes, if desired.
6. Best served fresh.

Nutrition: Calories: 536; Fat: 46g; Protein: 18g; Carbs: 18g; Fibre: 14g

FRENCH TOAST STICKS

5 minutes   10 minutes   6

INGREDIENTS

- 3 tbsp. of caster sugar
- Salt
- 80 ml of double cream
- 1/4 tsp. of ground cinnamon
- 1/2 tsp. of vanilla extract
- 6 thick slices white loaf or brioche, each slice cut into thirds
- Maple syrup, for serving
- 2 large eggs
- 80 ml of whole milk

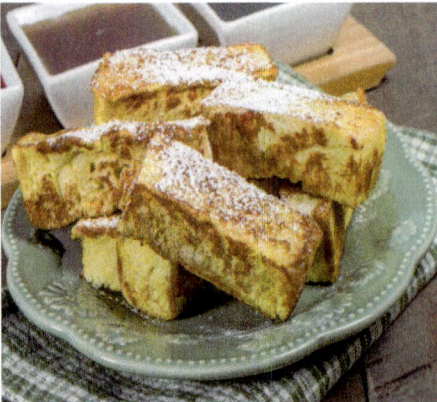

DIRECTIONS

1. Take a large shallow baking dish and beat sugar, cream, eggs, cinnamon, vanilla, milk, and a pinch of salt.
2. Add bread, turn to coat for few times.
3. Arrange the french toast into the Air Fryer basket, working in batches to not overcrowd the basket. Set Air Fryer to 190°C, cook until golden, about 8 minutes, tossing halfway through.
4. Serve warm, drizzled with maple syrup.

Nutrition: Calories: 166; Fat: 7 g; Protein: 6 g; Carbs: 18 g; Fibre: 2.5 g; Sugar: 7 g

SAUSAGES IN AIR FRYER

5 minutes

12 minutes

6

INGREDIENTS

- 6 Sausages
- 3 squirts Spray Oil

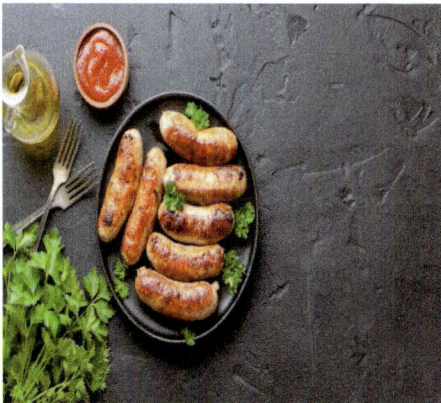

DIRECTIONS

1. Preheat your air fryer to 180°C for 5 minutes
2. Prick each sausage a couple of times (you can use a knife or fork).
3. Spray the bottom of the air fryer with a few splashes of oil to prevent the sausages from sticking.
4. Use the tongs to gently insert the sausages (do not let them touch so that they cook evenly).
5. Set timer to 12 minutes (adjust the time for small, large or frozen sausages).
6. Halfway through cooking, turn with tongs.
7. Check after 12 minutes and reheat if necessary. Serve with your chosen meal

Nutrition: Calories: 209; Carbs: 2g; Protein: 11g; Fat: 17g

FRIED BACON

10 minutes   10 minutes   2

INGREDIENTS

- 4-5 rashers of lean bacon, fat cut off

DIRECTIONS

1. Line up the Air Fryer basket with parchment paper, to soak up excess grease
2. Arrange your bacon in the basket, ensuring you don't overcrowd; around 4-5 slices should be enough, depending upon the size of your machine
3. Set the fryer to 200°C
4. Cook for 10 minutes for crispy, and an extra 2 if you want it super-crispy
5. Serve and enjoy!

Nutrition: Calories: 161; Fat: 12 g; Protein: 12 g; Carbs: 0.5 g; Fibre: 0 g; Sugar: 0 g

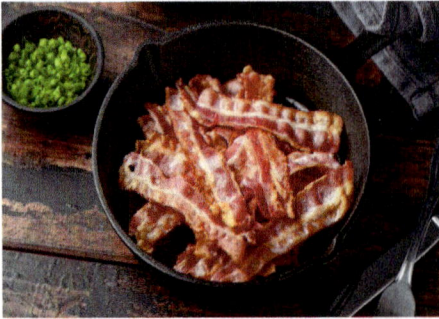

BLT BREAKFAST WRAP

5 minutes | 10 minutes | 4

INGREDIENTS

- 227 g reduced-sodium bacon
- 8 tbsp mayonnaise
- 8 large romaine lettuce leaves
- 4 Roma tomatoes, sliced
- Salt and ground black pepper, to taste

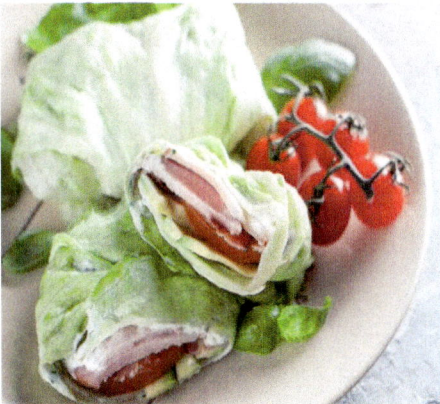

DIRECTIONS

1. Set the bacon in a single layer in the air fryer basket. (It's OK if the bacon sits a bit on the sides.) Set the air fryer to 177C and air fry for 10 min. Check for crispiness and air fry for 2 to 3 min longer if needed. Cook in batches, if necessary, and drain the grease in between sets.
2. Scatter 1 tbsp of mayonnaise on each of the lettuce leaves and top with the tomatoes and cooked bacon. Flavour to taste with salt and freshly ground black pepper.
3. Roll the lettuce leaves as you would a burrito, securing with a toothpick if desired.

Nutrition: Calories: 370 Fat: 34g; Protein: 11g Carbs: 7g; Fibre: 3g

BOILED EGGS IN AIR FRYER

1 minutes

10 minutes

4

INGREDIENTS

- 4 eggs (use as many as you want)

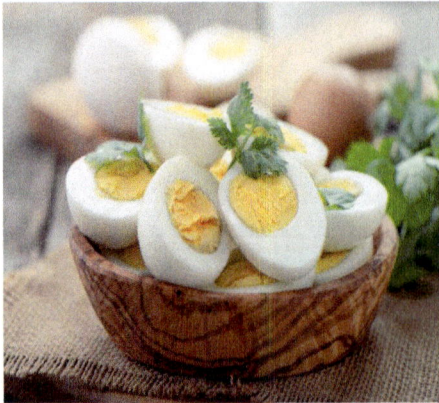

DIRECTIONS

1. Place room temperature eggs in the basket of the air fryer, leaving space between the eggs to allow the hot air to circulate. Use a metal rack to fit more, if necessary.
2. Set the air fryer to 150°C. Cook according to your preferences (from 8 minutes for soft-boiled eggs to 12 minutes for hard-boiled eggs).
3. Once cooked, remove from the air fryer basket and place in an ice bath or bowl of cold water. This will prevent the eggs from continuing to cook. When it's cool and safe to touch, remove the skin.

Nutrition: Calories: 72; Fat: 5g; Carbs: 0g; Fibre: 0g; Sugar: 0g; Protein: 6g

CHOCOLATE PUDDING

15 minutes

10 minutes

2

INGREDIENTS

- 60 ml of butter
- 60 ml of whole milk
- 120 grams of chocolate chips, melted
- 1 egg
- 4 tablespoons of sugar
- Spray oil, for greasing
- 240g of flour

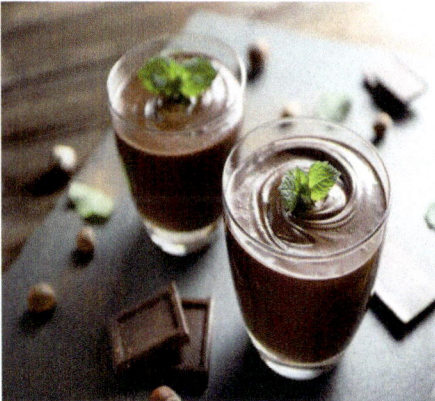

DIRECTIONS

1. Take a bowl and put the butter in it.
2. Melt it by putting it in the microwave.
3. Mix well and add the sugar and milk.
4. At the end, add egg and flour.
5. Incorporate the melted chocolate chips.
6. Pour this mixture into greased molds.
7. Place the molds in the basket of the air fryer and cook for 10 minutes at 40 degs C.
8. When ready, serve and enjoy.
9. The internal consistency will be liquid.

Nutrition: Calories: 800; Fat: 46 g; Protein: 31 g; Carbs: 64 g; Fibre: 4 g; Sugar: 36 g

CHAPTER 2: MAIN DISH RECIPES

FRIED RICE

10 minutes   20 minutes   4

INGREDIENTS

- 300g chicken tenderloins
- 4 rashers rindless bacon
- 450g packet microwave long-grain rice
- 2 tbsp oyster sauce
- 2 tbsp light soy sauce
- 1 tsp sesame oil
- 3 tsp finely grated fresh ginger
- 2 eggs, lightly whisked
- 120g (3/4 cup) frozen peas
- 2 green shallots, sliced
- 1 long fresh red chilli, thinly sliced
- Oyster sauce, to drizzle

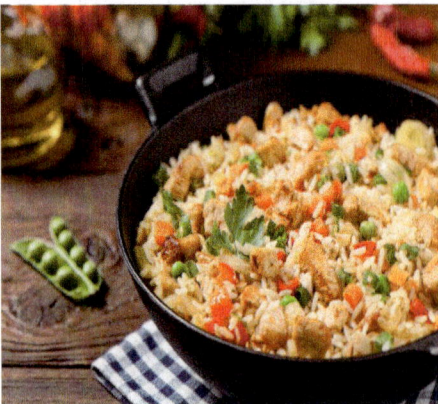

DIRECTIONS

1. Preheat the air fryer to 180C. Place the chicken and bacon on the air fryer rack. Cook for 8 minutes or until cooked through. Transfer to a plate and set aside to cool slightly. Slice the chicken and chop the bacon.
2. Meanwhile, use your fingers to separate the rice grains in the packet. Microwave the rice for 1 minute. Transfer to a round 20cm, high-sided ovenproof dish or cake pan. Add the oyster sauce, soy sauce, sesame oil, ginger and 2 tablespoons water. Stir to combine.
3. Place the dish or pan in the air fryer. Cook for 5 minutes or until the rice is tender. Stir through the egg, peas , chicken and half of the bacon. Cook for 3 minutes or until the egg is cooked through. Stir in half the shallot and season with salt and white pepper.
4. Serve sprinkled with chilli, remaining shallot, remaining bacon and extra oyster sauce.

Nutrition: Calories: 554; Fat: 7 g; Protein: 24 g; Carbs: 92 g; Fibre: 3 g; Sugar: 1 g

VEGETARIAN PUMPKIN SCHNITZEL

30 minutes   30 minutes   2

INGREDIENTS

- 500g potatoes, peeled, cut into 3-4cm pieces
- 250g swede or turnip, peeled, cut into 3-4cm pieces
- 2 1/2 tbsp extra virgin olive oil
- 1/2 cup Panko breadcrumbs
- 1/4 cup finely grated cheddar
- 2 tbsp finely chopped hazelnuts
- 1 tbsp finely chopped flat-leaf parsley, plus extra to serve
- 500g butternut pumpkin, peeled
- 1 egg
- Lemon wedges, to serve

DIRECTIONS

1. Place potatoes and turnip in a medium saucepan and cover with water. Season with salt. Bring to the boil over high heat. Gently boil, covered, for 15 minutes or until tender. Drain well and return to pan. Add 2 tablespoons oil and mash until smooth. Season with salt and pepper.
2. Meanwhile, Preheat the Air fryer to 180C.
3. Combine breadcrumbs, cheddar, hazelnuts, parsley and remaining oil in a shallow dish. Season with salt and pepper. Cut pumpkin into 1cm thick slices. Lightly beat egg on a shallow plate.
4. Dip pumpkin into egg to cover all over. Press into breadcrumb mixture to coat all over. Place in the basket, using the grill separator to arrange a second layer of pumpkin. Insert basket into Air fryer. Cook for 12 minutes or until golden and tender.
5. Serve pumpkin schnitzels with mash and lemon wedges. Sprinkle with extra chopped parsley.

Nutrition: Calories: 650; Fat: 24.5 g; Protein: 18.5 g; Carbs: 87 g; Fibre: 9 g; Sugar: 14.5 g

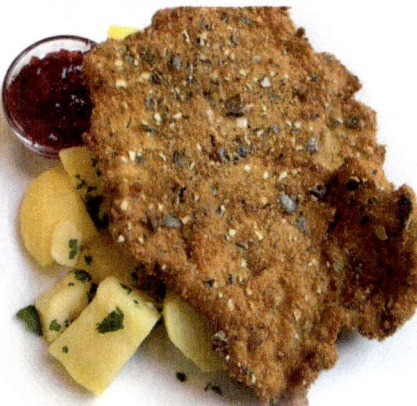

DORITOS-CRUMBED CHICKEN TENDERS

4h 15 minutes

20 minutes

4

INGREDIENTS

- 500g chicken tenderloins, halved crossways
- 250ml (1 cup) buttermilk
- 170g packet Doritos Nacho Cheese corn chips
- 1 egg, lightly whisked
- 50g (1/3 cup) plain flour
- Mild salsa, to serve

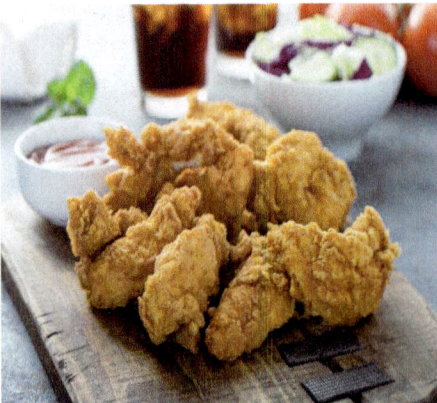

DIRECTIONS

1. Place the chicken in a glass or ceramic bowl. Cover with the buttermilk. Cover and place in the fridge for 4 hours or overnight to marinate.
2. Preheat an air fryer to 180C. Line a baking tray with baking paper.
3. Place the corn chips in a food processor and pulse until coarsely chopped. Transfer to a plate. Place the egg in a shallow bowl. Place the flour on a separate plate.
4. Drain the chicken, discarding the buttermilk. Dip the chicken in the flour and shake off excess. Dip in the egg then in corn chips, pressing firmly to coat. Transfer to the prepared tray.
5. Place half the chicken in the air fryer and fry for 8-10 minutes or until golden and cooked through. Repeat with remaining chicken tenders.
6. Transfer to a serving platter. Serve with salsa.

Nutrition: Calories: 468; Fat: 15.5 g; Protein: 46 g; Carbs: 33 g; Fibre: 1 g; Sugar: 24.5 g

CHICKEN NUGGETS

20 minutes   10 minutes   4

INGREDIENTS

- 500g chicken tenders
- 4 tbsp. salad dressing mix
- 2 tbsp. plain flour
- 1 egg, beaten
- 50g dry breadcrumbs

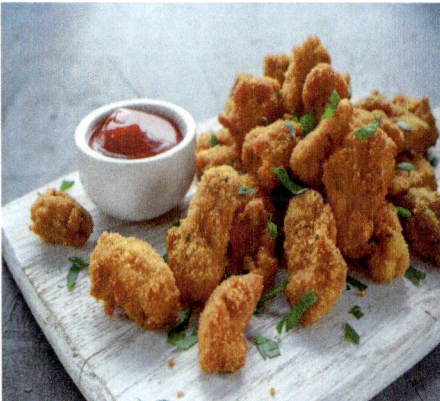

DIRECTIONS

1. Take a large mixing bowl and add the chicken
2. Sprinkle the seasoning over the top and ensure the chicken is evenly coated
3. Allow the chicken to rest for 10 minutes
4. Add the flour into a resealable bag
5. Pour the breadcrumbs onto a medium sized plate
6. Transfer the chicken into the resealable bag and coat with the flour, giving it a good shake
7. Remove the chicken and dip into the egg, and then roll into the breadcrumbs, coating evenly
8. Repeat with the chicken
9. Heat your Air Fryer to 200°C
10. Arrange the chicken inside the fryer and cook for 4 minutes, before turning over and cooking for another 4 minutes
11. Remove and serve whilst hot

Nutrition: Calories: 291.5; Fat: 13 g; Protein: 29 g; Carbs: 11 g; Fibre: 1 g; Sugar: 0.5 g

CHICKEN PARMESAN IN AIR FRYER

10 minutes   14 minutes   4

INGREDIENTS

- 2 large boneless chicken breasts
- Salt
- Freshly ground black pepper
- 40 g plain flour
- 2 large eggs
- 100 g panko breadcrumbs
- 25 g freshly grated Parmesan
- 1 tsp. dried oregano
- 1/2 tsp. garlic powder
- 1/2 tsp. chilli flakes
- 240 g marinara/tomato sauce
- 100 g grated mozzarella
- Freshly chopped parsley, for garnish

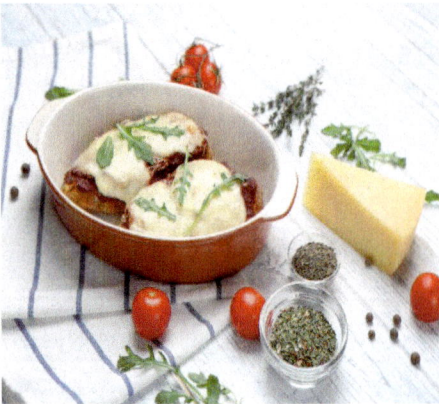

DIRECTIONS

1. Gently butterfly the chicken, cutting in half width wise to obtain 4 thin chicken pieces. Season with salt and pepper on both sides.
2. Place the flour in a shallow bowl and season with a large pinch of salt and pepper. Put the eggs in a second bowl and beat them. In a third bowl, mix together the breadcrumbs, parmesan cheese, oregano, garlic powder, and chilli flakes.
3. Working with chicken pieces one at a time, coat them in flour, then dip them in the eggs and finally press them into the panko mixture, being careful to coat both sides well.
4. Working in batches as needed, place the chicken in the basket and air fry at 200°C for 5 minutes per side. Top chicken with sauce and mozzarella and cook at 200°C for a further 3 minutes or until cheese is melted and golden.
5. Garnish with parsley to serve.

Nutrition: Calories: 419.5; Fat: 16 g; Protein: 30 g; Carbs: 32 g; Fibre: 3 g; Sugar: 10 g

TURKEY AND MUSHROOM BURGERS

10 minutes   10 minutes   2

INGREDIENTS

- 180g mushrooms
- 500g minced turkey
- 1 tsp. garlic powder
- 1 tsp. onion powder
- ½ tsp. salt
- ½ tsp. pepper

DIRECTIONS

1. Take your food processor and add the mushrooms, pulsing into they form a puree. Season and pulse once more
2. Remove from the food processor and tip into a mixing bowl
3. Add the turkey to the bowl and combine well
4. Take a little of the mixture into your hands and shape into burgers. You should be able to make five
5. Spray each burger with a little cooking spray and place in the Air Fryer
6. Cook at 160°C for 10 minutes

Nutrition: Calories: 357.5; Fat: 14 g; Protein: 54 g; Carbs: 0 g; Fibre: 0 g; Sugar: 0 g

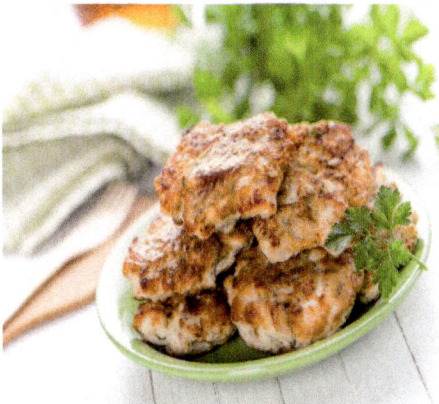

SPICY CHICKEN THIGHS

10 minutes   25 minutes   4

INGREDIENTS

- 80 ml low-sodium soy sauce
- Thinly sliced spring onions, for garnish
- 2 tbsp. chilli garlic sauce
- Juice of 1 lime
- Toasted sesame seeds, for garnish
- 2 cloves garlic, crushed
- 2 tsp. freshly grated ginger
- 60 ml extra-virgin olive oil
- 2 tbsp. honey
- 4 bone-in, skin-on chicken thighs

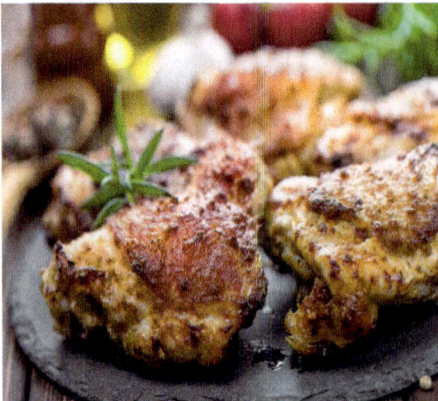

DIRECTIONS

1. Take a large bowl, mix oil, soy sauce, honey, garlic, chilli garlic sauce, lime juice, and ginger. Reserve a cup of 120ml of marinade. Add chicken thighs to the bowl and toss to coat. Now cover and refrigerate for 30 minutes or more.

2. Remove 2 of the thighs from the marinade and arrange them in the Air Fryer basket. Cook at 200°C until thighs are reach an internal temperature of 73°C, 15-20 minutes. Now transfer the thighs to a plate, tent with foil. Now repeat with the remaining thighs.

3. Meanwhile, take a small saucepan over medium heat, bring marinade to a boil. Reduce heat, simmer until sauce thickens slightly, 4-5 minutes.

4. Brush the sauce over the thighs, garnish with spring onions and sesame seeds.

Nutrition: Calories: 524; Fat: 48 g; Protein: 10 g; Carbs: 14 g; Fibre: 0.25 g; Sugar: 9 g

PESTO CHICKEN

10 minutes

20 minutes

2

INGREDIENTS

- 4 chicken drumsticks
- 6 garlic cloves
- 1/2 jalapeno pepper
- 2 tbsp. lemon juice
- 2 tbsp. olive oil
- 1 tbsp. ginger, sliced
- 65 grams coriander
- 1 tsp. salt

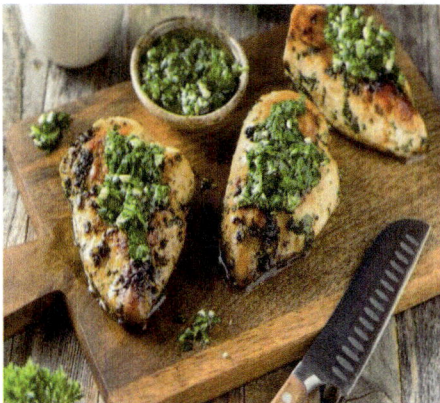

DIRECTIONS

1. Add all the ingredients except chicken into the blender and blend until smooth.
2. Pour blended mixture into a large bowl.
3. Add chicken and stir well to coat. Place in refrigerator for 2 hours.
4. Spray air fryer basket with cooking spray.
5. Place marinated chicken into the air fryer basket and cook at 200 degs C for 20 min. Turn halfway through.
6. Serve and enjoy.

Nutrition: Calories 305; Fat 19 g; Carbohydrates 5 g; Sugar 0.7 g; Protein 25 g

CHICKEN WINGS WITH HONEY AND SESAME

< 30 minutes

10-30 minutes

1-2

INGREDIENTS

- 450–500g chicken wings with tips removed
- 1 tbsp. olive oil
- 3 tbsp. cornflour
- 1 tbsp. runny honey
- 1 tsp. soy sauce or tamari
- 1 tsp. rice wine vinegar
- 1 tsp. toasted sesame oil
- 2 tsp. sesame seeds, toasted
- 1 large spring onion, thinly sliced
- salt and freshly ground black pepper

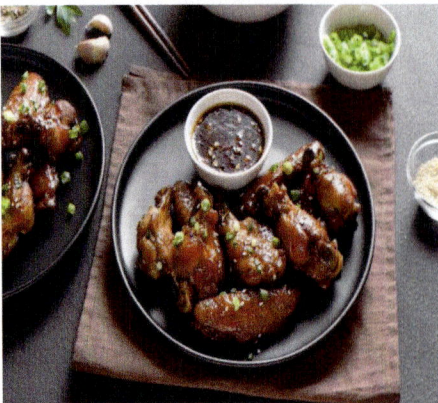

DIRECTIONS

1. Take a large bowl, toss together chicken wings, olive oil and a generous amount of salt and black pepper.
2. Toss in the cornflour, one tablespoon at a time, until the wings are well coated.
3. Air-fry the chicken wings in a single layer for 25 minutes, 180°C, turning halfway through.
4. Meanwhile, in a large bowl, make the glaze by whisking together the soy sauce, honey, rice, wine vinegar and toasted sesame oil.
5. Now tip the cooked wings into the glaze, tossing until coated. Place them in the Air Fryer in a single layer for another 5 minutes.
6. Toss the wings in the remaining glaze. Now sprinkle with the toasted sesame seeds and the spring onion.
7. Serve.

Nutrition: Calories: 544; Fat: 32.5 g; Protein: 37.5g; Carbs: 23.5 g; Fibre: 2 g; Sugar: 9 g

CHICKEN BREAST

5 minutes

15 minutes

2

INGREDIENTS

- Wax paper or plastic wrap
- 2 skinless/boneless chicken breast halves
- 1 tsp. salt
- 2 tsp. paprika
- 2 tsp. onion powder
- 2 tsp. black pepper
- 1 tsp. white pepper
- 1 tsp. cayenne pepper
- 1 tsp. ground cumin
- 1 tsp. ground oregano

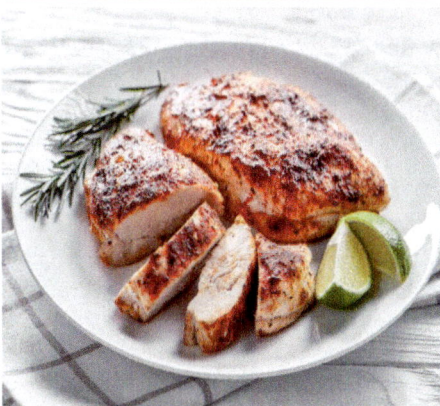

DIRECTIONS

1. Put your chicken breasts between a few sheets of wax paper or plastic wrap and use a meat pounder until the chicken is evenly thick.
2. Make the blackened seasoning by mixing paprika, salt, onion powder, the 3 types of pepper, ground cumin, ground oregano. Check that the spices are well mixed.
3. Dredge the chicken in the seasoning spice mixture.
4. Place the chicken breasts in the Air Fryer basket. Temperature to 145°C, cook for 8 minutes.
5. After 8 minutes, remove the basket, turn the chicken breasts over. Set the temperature to 180°C and cook for 6 more minutes.

Nutrition: Calories: 355.5; Fat: 18.5 g; Protein: 41.5 g; Carbs: 1 g; Fibre: 0 g; Sugar: 0 g

CHICKEN STRIPS

< 30 minutes   10-30 minutes   3

INGREDIENTS

- 2 large garlic cloves, minced or crushed
- 5 tbsp. plain yogurt
- ¼ tsp. salt, plus extra for seasoning
- 2 chicken breasts
- 6 tbsp. plain flour
- 6 tbsp. panko breadcrumbs
- 1 tsp. sweet smoked paprika
- 1 tsp. garlic granules
- ½ tsp. cayenne pepper
- freshly ground black pepper
- 1 free-range egg
- olive oil cooking spray

For the creamy honey mustard dip:

- 1 tbsp. runny honey
- 1 tbsp. light mayonnaise
- 1 tbsp. Dijon mustard
- ½ tbsp. wholegrain mustard
- ½ tsp. white wine vinegar

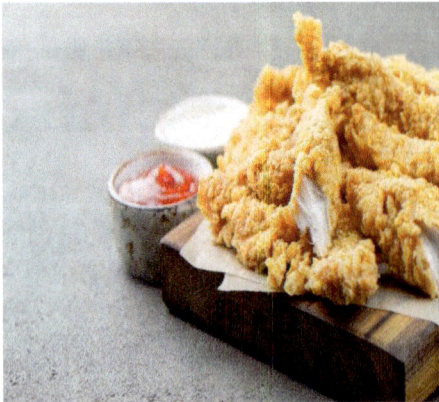

DIRECTIONS

1. To marinate the chicken, mix garlic, yoghurt and salt. Cut the chicken into 3cm wide strips, marinate in the yoghurt mixture for 20 minutes or more.
2. Take a medium bowl and mix the flour, paprika, breadcrumbs, cayenne pepper, garlic granules and a good amount of salt and pepper to create dredging mixture. Take another small bowl, beat the egg and add salt, pepper.
3. Shake off any excess yogurt from each of the chicken strip before dipping it first in the egg, then in the dredging mixture. Use different hands for wet and dry ingredients.
4. Spray the bottom of the Air Fryer basket with olive oil spray, arrange a single layer of chicken strips in the bottom. Spray the top of the strips with oil before air-frying 15 minutes, 200°C, turning roughly halfway through. Repeat until all the strips are cooked (work in batches).
5. Meanwhile, mix all the ingredients for the creamy honey mustard dip in a small bowl, set aside.
6. Serve.

Nutrition: Calories: 452; Fat: 15.5 g; Protein: 36 g; Carbs: 38 g; Fibre: 3 g; Sugar: 2.5 g

HERBED STEAK

30 minutes

20 minutes

4

INGREDIENTS

- 4 tbsp. butter, softened
- 2 cloves garlic, crushed
- 2 tsp. freshly chopped parsley
- 1 tsp. freshly chopped chives
- 1 tsp. freshly chopped thyme
- 1 tsp. freshly chopped rosemary
- 1 (900g) bone-in ribeye
- Salt
- Freshly ground black pepper

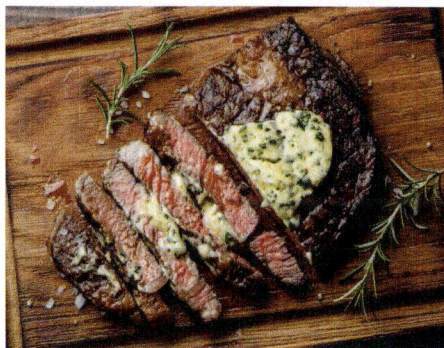

DIRECTIONS

1. In a small bowl, mix butter, herbs. Arrange in centre of a piece of cling film and roll into a log. Twist ends together to keep tight and refrigerate until hardened, 20 minutes.
2. Add salt and pepper on both sides of the steak.
3. Place steak in the Air Fryer basket and cook, flipping halfway through, 200°C 12-14 minutes for medium, depending on thickness of steak.
4. Top your steak with a slice of herb butter.

Nutrition: Calories: 415; Fat: 22 g; Protein: 51 g; Carbs: 3 g; Fibre: 0 g; Sugar: 0 g

TERIYAKI PORK AND MUSHROOM ROLLS

10 minutes   8 minutes   6

INGREDIENTS

- 4 tbsp brown sugar
- 4 tbsp mirin
- 4 tbsp soy sauce
- 1 tsp almond flour
- 5 cm ginger, chopped
- 452 grams of pork belly slices
- 170 grams of Enoki mushrooms

DIRECTIONS

1. Mix the brown sugar, mirin, soy sauce, almond flour, and ginger together until brown sugar dissolves.
2. Take pork belly slices and wrap around a bundle of mushrooms. Brush each roll with teriyaki sauce. Chill for half an hour.
3. Place the crisper tray on the air fry position. Select Air Fry, set the temperature to 177 degs C and set the time to 8 min.
4. Add marinated pork rolls to the crisper tray.
5. Air fry for 8 min. Flip the rolls halfway through.
6. Serve immediately.

Nutrition: Calories 97; Fat 9 g; Carbohydrates 2.2 g; Protein 2 g; Fibre: 0.6 g; Sugar 6 g

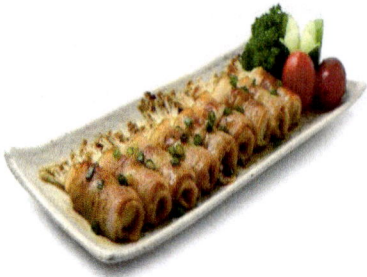

PORK CHOPS

10 minutes   10 minutes   4

INGREDIENTS

- 4 boneless pork chops
- 2 tbsp. extra-virgin olive oil
- 50 g freshly grated Parmesan
- 1 tsp. salt
- 1 tsp. paprika
- 1 tsp. garlic powder
- 1 tsp. onion powder
- 1/2 tsp. freshly ground black pepper

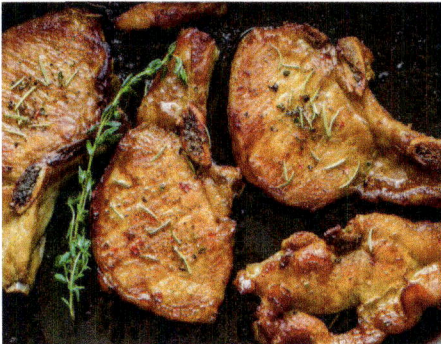

DIRECTIONS

1. Pat your pork chops dry with some paper towels, then coat both of the sides with oil. Take a medium bowl, mix Parmesan, spices. Coat both of the sides of the pork chops with the Parmesan mixture.
2. Place the pork chops in Air Fryer basket, cook at 190°C for 9 minutes, flipping halfway through.

Nutrition: Calories: 306; Fat: 22 g; Protein: 23 g; Carbs: 1.5 g; Fibre: 0 g; Sugar: 0 g

BALSAMIC LONDON BROIL

15 minutes   25 minutes   8

INGREDIENTS

- 900 grams of London broil
- 3 large garlic cloves, minced
- 3 tbsp balsamic vinegar
- 3 tbsp whole-grain mustard
- 2 tbsp olive oil
- Sea salt and ground black pepper, to taste
- 1/2 tsps dried hot red pepper flakes

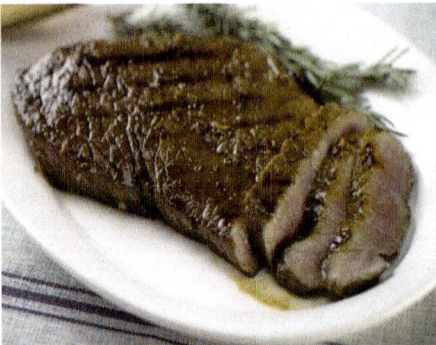

DIRECTIONS

1. Wash and dry the London broil. Score the sides with a knife.
2. Mix the remaining ingredients. Rub this mixture onto the broil, coating it well. Allow marinating for a minimum of 3 hours.
3. Place the crisper tray on the air fry position. Select Air Fry, set the temperature to 200 degs C and set the time to 25 min.
4. Place the meat in the crisper tray. Air fry for 15 min. Turn it over and air fry for an additional 10 min before serving.

Nutrition: Calories 198; Fat 6.2 g; Carbohydrates 0.7 g; Protein 35 g; Fibre: 0.25 g; Sugar 0.1 g

BEEF WELLINGTON

15 minutes

35 minutes

8

INGREDIENTS

- 1kg beef fillet (one large piece)
- Chicken pate
- 2 sheets of shortcrust pastry
- 1 egg, beaten
- Salt
- Pepper

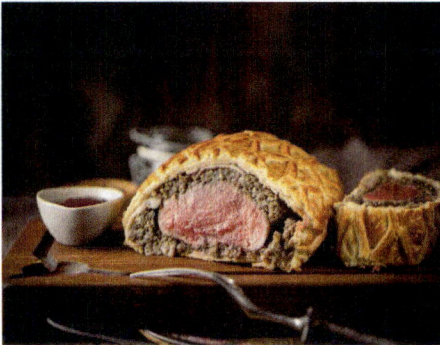

DIRECTIONS

1. Season the beef with salt, pepper and wrap tightly in cling film
2. Place the beef in the refrigerator for at least one hour
3. Roll out the pastry and brush the edges with the beaten egg
4. Spread the pate over the pastry, making sure it is distributed equally
5. Take now the beef out of the refrigerator and remove the cling film
6. Place the beef in the middle of your pastry
7. Wrap your pastry around the meat and seal the edges with a fork
8. Place in the Air Fryer and cook at 160°C for 35 minutes

Nutrition: Calories: 509; Fat: 28 g; Protein: 34 g; Carbs: 28 g; Fibre: 1 g; Sugar: 0.5 g

PORK, SQUASH, AND PEPPER KEBABS

1 hour 20 minutes   8 minutes   4

INGREDIENTS

For the Pork:

- 450 grams of pork steak, cut into cubes
- 1 tbsp white wine vinegar
- 3 tbsp steak sauce
- 32 grams soy sauce
- 1 tsp powdered chili
- 1 tsp red chili flakes
- 2 tsps smoked paprika
- 1 tsp garlic salt

For the Vegetable:

- 1 green squash, deseeded and cut into cubes
- 1 yellow squash, deseeded and cut into cubes
- 1 red pepper, cut into cubes
- 1 green pepper, cut into cubes
- Salt and ground black pepper, to taste
- Cooking Spray

Special Equipment:

- 4 bamboo skewers, soaked in water for at least 30 min

DIRECTIONS

1. Combine the ingredients for the pork in a large bowl. Dip the pork in the marinade. Wrap the bowl in plastic and let it rest in the refrigerator for at least an hour.
2. Spritz the air fry basket with cooking spray.
3. Remove the pork from the marinade and run the skewers through the pork and vegetables alternatively. Sprinkle with salt and pepper to taste.
4. Arrange the skewers in the basket and spritz with cooking spray.
5. Place the basket on the air fry position.
6. Select Air Fry. Set temperature to 193 degs C and set time to 8 min.
7. After 4 min, remove the basket from the air fryer grill. Flip the skewers. Return the basket to the air fryer grill and continue cooking.
8. When cooking is complete, the pork should be browned, and the vegetables should be lightly charred and tender.
9. Serve immediately.

Nutrition: Calories 240; Fat 13.5 g; Carbohydrates 5 g; Protein 20 g; Fibre: 0.8 g; Sugar 3 g

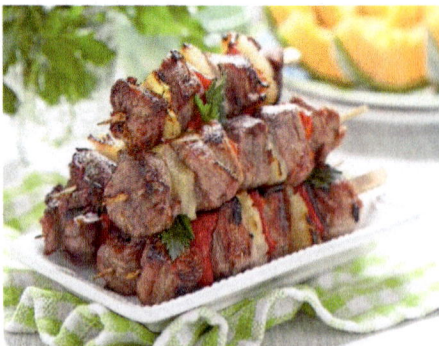

LAMB STEAKS

5 minutes

10 minutes

4

INGREDIENTS

- 4 Lamb Steaks
- 1 tsp. Frozen Chopped Garlic
- 2 tsp. Extra Virgin Olive Oil
- 2 tsp. Lemon Juice
- 2 tsp. Honey
- 1 tsp. Thyme
- Salt & Pepper
- Fresh Mint

DIRECTIONS

1. Place the lamb steaks on a chopping board, season with salt, pepper and dried thyme.
2. Thinly chop two tablespoons of mint and load into a bowl with everything except the lamb. Mix well then spoon over the lamb steaks. Place the steaks into the fridge for an hour, allow to marinate.
3. Put the steaks into the Air Fryer basket, add extra mint.
4. Air fry 10 minutes, 180°C.

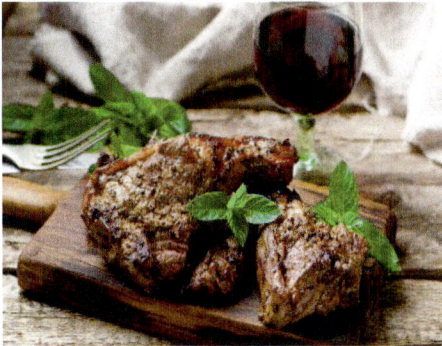

Nutrition: Calories: 274.5; Fat: 19 g; Protein: 21g; Carbs: 4 g; Fibre: 0 g; Sugar: 4 g

SIMPLE HAMBURGERS

5 minutes

15 minutes

4

INGREDIENTS

- 500 g minced beef
- Salt
- Pepper

DIRECTIONS

1. Preheat Air Fryer to 200°C.
2. Divide minced beef into 4 equal portions and form them into burgers with your hands.
3. Season with salt, pepper, to your taste.
4. Air fry for 10 minutes.
5. Flip your burgers over, cook for a further 3 minutes.

Nutrition: Calories: 247.5; Fat: 15 g; Protein: 24 g; Carbs: 0 g; Fibre: 0 g; Sugar: 0 g

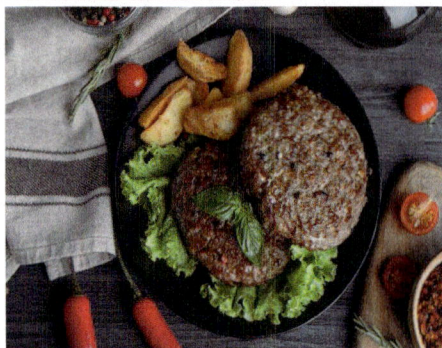

CRAB CAKES

20 minutes   15 minutes   4

INGREDIENTS

For The Crab Cakes:

- Cooking spray
- Hot sauce, for serving
- Lemon wedges, for serving
- 60 g of mayonnaise
- 1 egg
- 2 tsp. of cajun seasoning
- 1 tsp. of lemon zest
- 1/2 tsp. of salt
- 450 g of jumbo lump crab meat
- 120 g of Cracker crumbs (from about 20 crackers)
- 2 tbsp. of chives, finely chopped
- 2 tsp. of Dijon mustard

For The Tartar Sauce:

- 1/4 tsp. of Dijon mustard
- 1 tsp. of fresh dill, finely chopped
- 60 g of mayonnaise
- 80 g dill pickle, finely chopped
- 2 tsp. of capers, finely chopped
- 1 tsp. of fresh lemon juice
- 1 tbsp. of shallot, finely chopped

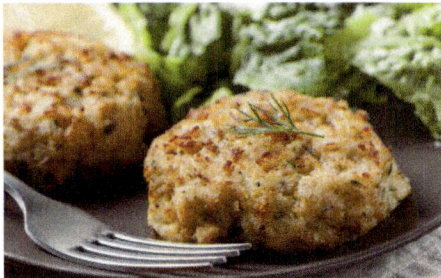

DIRECTIONS

1 Take a large bowl, whisk together egg, mayo, chives, Dijon mustard, lemon zest, cajun seasoning, and salt. Fold in crab meat and cracker crumbs.
2 Divide your mixture to form 8 patties.
3 Heat your Air Fryer to 190°C, spray the basket and the tops of your cakes with some cooking spray. Arrange the cakes into the basket in a single layer. Cook until crisp and deep golden brown, 12-14 minutes, flip halfway through.
4 Take a bowl and mix all of the tartar sauce ingredients.
5 Serve the cakes warm with lemon wedges, hot sauce and tartar sauce.

Nutrition: Calories: 265; Fat: 8 g; Protein: 24.5 g; Carbs: 21 g; Fibre: 1 g; Sugar: 0 g

FISH TACOS

14 minutes   10 minutes   4

INGREDIENTS

- 500g mahi fish, fresh
- 8 small tortillas
- 2 tsp. Cajun seasoning
- 4 tbsp. sour cream
- 2 tbsp. mayo
- ¼ tbsp. cayenne
- 2 tbsp. pepper sauce
- A little salt and pepper
- 1 tbsp. sriracha sauce
- 2 tbsp. lime juice

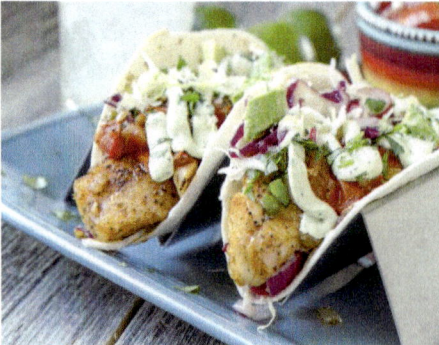

DIRECTIONS

1 Cut the fish into slices and season with salt
2 Mix the cayenne pepper and black pepper with the Cajun seasoning. Sprinkle onto fish
3 Brush pepper sauce on both sides of the fish
4 Set Air Fryer to 180°C and cook for 10 mins
5 Take a medium bowl and combine the mayonnaise, sour cream, lime juice, sriracha and cayenne pepper
6 Assemble the tacos and serve!

Nutrition: Calories: 447; Fat: 13 g; Protein: 31 g; Carbs: 48 g; Fibre: 3 g; Sugar: 3.5 g

SALMON FILLET IN AIR FRYER

10 minutes

15 minutes

4

INGREDIENTS

- 2 salmon fillets
- 1/2 tbsp olive oil
- Salt and pepper to season

DIRECTIONS

1. Turn on your air fryer and set the temperature to 200°C.
2. Brush each salmon fillet with a little oil and season with salt and pepper or your favourite seasoning/marinade.
3. Lightly spray the air fryer basket with oil and place the salmon fillets in the basket. Air Fry for 8 minutes. At this point, check to see if they are done. Heat for an additional 1-2 minutes, if necessary.

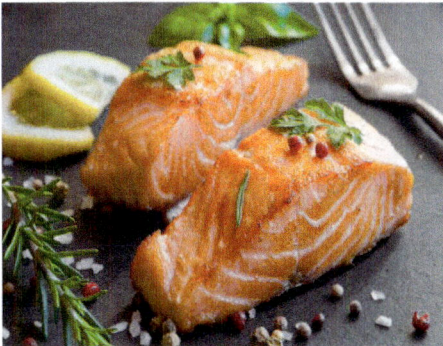

Nutrition: Calories: 310.5; Fat: 15.5 g; Protein: 39 g; Carbs: 0 g; Fibre: 0 g; Sugar: 0 g

FRIED COD

15 minutes   15 minutes   3

INGREDIENTS

- 1 (450g) cod, cut into 4 strips
- Salt
- Freshly ground black pepper
- 65 g plain flour
- 1 large egg, beaten
- 200 g panko breadcrumbs
- 1 tsp. Old Bay seasoning
- Lemon wedges, for serving
- Tartar sauce, for serving

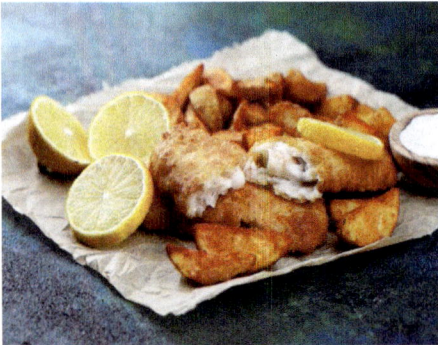

DIRECTIONS

1   Pat the fish dry and add salt and pepper on both sides.
2   Arrange egg, flour, and panko in three shallow bowls. Add Old Bay to panko and toss. Coat fish into the flour, then into the egg, and finally into panko, press to coat, one at a time.
3   Arrange the fish into the Air Fryer basket, cook 10-12 minutes, 200°C, or until fish is golden and flakes easily with a fork, gently flip halfway through.
4   Serve with lemon wedges and tartar sauce.

Nutrition: Calories: 397; Fat: 4.5 g; Protein: 37 g; Carbs: 48 g; Fibre: 3.5 g; Sugar: 3.5 g

BEERY COD FILLET

5 minutes   15 minutes   4

INGREDIENTS

- 2 eggs
- 130 grams malty beer
- 130 grams all-purpose flour
- 65 grams cornstarch
- 1 tsp garlic powder
- Salt and pepper, to taste
- 450 grams of cod fillets
- Cooking Spray

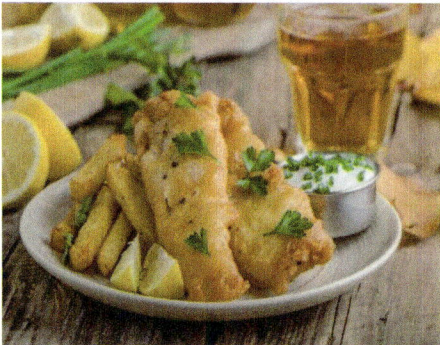

DIRECTIONS

1. In a shallow bowl, beat together the eggs with the beer. In another shallow bowl, thoroughly combine the cornstarch and flour. Sprinkle with salt, garlic powder, and pepper.
2. Dredge each cod fillet in the flour mixture, then in the egg mixture. Dip each piece of fish in the flour mixture a second time.
3. Spritz the air fry basket with cooking spray. Arrange the cod fillets in the basket in a single layer.
4. Place the basket on the air fry position.
5. Select Air Fry, set the temperature to 200 degs C, and set time to 15 min. Flip the fillets halfway through the Cooking.
6. When cooking is complete, the cod should reach an internal temperature of 63 degs C on a meat thermometer and the outside should be crispy. Let the fish cool for 5 min and serve.

Nutrition: Calories 310; Fat 4.8 g; Carbs 33.8 g; Protein 30 g; Fibre: 33.8 g; Sugar 0 g

SHRIMP SALAD WITH CAESAR DRESSING

10 minutes   15 minutes   4

INGREDIENTS

- ½ baguette, cut into 2.5 cm cubes (about 264 grams)
- 4 tbsp extra-virgin olive oil, divided
- ¼ tsp granulated garlic
- ¼ tsp kosher salt
- 95 grams Caesar dressing, divided
- 2 romaine lettuce hearts, cut in half lengthwise and ends trimmed
- 455 grams of medium shrimp, peeled and deveined
- 60 grams of Parmesan cheese, coarsely grated

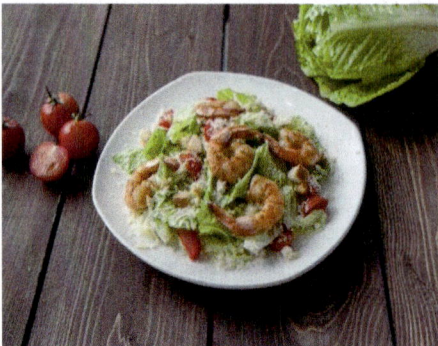

DIRECTIONS

1. Make the croutons: Put the bread cubes in a medium bowl and drizzle 3 tbsp of olive oil over top. Season with salt and granulated garlic and toss to coat. Transfer to the air fry basket in a single layer.
2. Place the basket on the air fry position.
3. Select Air Fry, set temperature to 200 degs C, and set time to 4 min. Toss the croutons halfway through the cooking.
4. When done, remove the air fry basket from the air fryer grill and set aside.
5. Brush 2 tbsp of Caesar dressing on the cut side of the lettuce. Set aside.
6. Toss the shrimp with the 32 grams of Caesar dressing in a large bowl until well coated. Set aside.
7. Coat the sheet pan with the remaining 1 tbsp of olive oil. Arrange the romaine halves on the coated pan, cut side down. Brush the tops with the remaining 2 tbsp of Caesar dressing.
8. Place the pan on the toast position.
9. Select Toast, set temperature to 190 degs C, and set time to 10 min.
10. After 5 min, remove the pan from the air fryer grill and flip the romaine halves. Spoon the shrimp around the lettuce. Return the pan to the air fryer grill and continue cooking.
11. When done, remove the sheet pan from the air fryer grill. If they are not quite cooked through, roast for another 1 minute.
12. On each of four plates, put a romaine half. Divide the shrimp among the plates and top with croutons and grated Parmesan cheese. Serve immediately.

Nutrition: Calories 286; Fat 17.5 g; Carbs 6.8 g; Protein 25.5 g; Fibre: 0.8 g; Sugar 0.3 g

PEPPERY LEMON SHRIMP

10 minutes

10 minutes

2

INGREDIENTS

- 1 tbsp. olive oil
- 350g prepared shrimps, uncooked
- Juice of 1 lemon
- 1 tsp. pepper
- ¼ tsp. paprika
- ¼ tsp. garlic powder
- 1 lemon, sliced

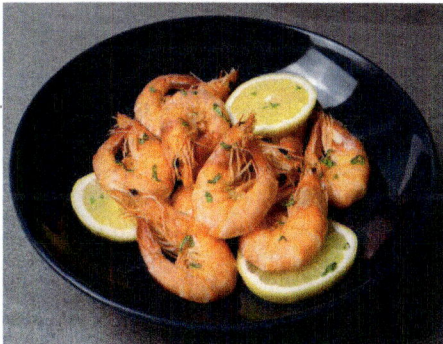

DIRECTIONS

1 Preheat the fryer to 200°C
2 Take a medium size mixing bowl, mix the pepper, lemon juice, garlic powder, paprika and the olive oil together
3 Add the shrimp to the bowl and make sure they're well coated
4 Arrange the shrimp into the basket of the fryer
5 Cook for between 6-8 minutes, until firm and pink
6 Serve!

Nutrition: Calories: 208; Fat: 7 g; Protein: 35 g; Carbs: 0 g; Fibre: 0 g; Sugar: 0 g

GOLD SALMON PATTIES

5 minutes

13 minutes

6 patties

INGREDIENTS

- 420 grams of can pink salmon, drained and bones removed
- 65 grams breadcrumbs
- 1 egg, whisked
- 2 scallions, diced
- 1 tsp garlic powder
- Salt and pepper, to taste
- Cooking Spray

DIRECTIONS

1. Stir together the salmon, breadcrumbs, whisked egg, garlic powder, scallions, salt, and pepper in a large bowl until well incorporated.
2. Divide the salmon mixture into six equal portions and form each into a patty with your hands.
3. Arrange the salmon patties in the air fry basket and spritz them with cooking spray.
4. Place the basket on the air fry position.
5. Air Fry, set the temperature to 200 degs C, and set time to 12 min. Flip the patties once halfway through.
6. When cooking is complete, the patties should be golden brown and cooked through. Remove the patties from the air fryer grill and serve on a plate.

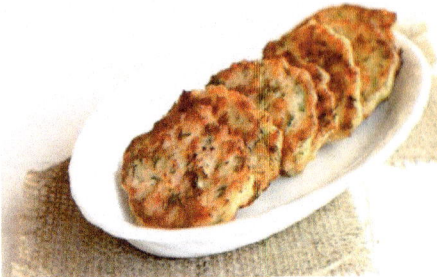

Nutrition: Calories 142; Fat 7.8 g; Carbohydrates 9.5 g; Protein 23 g; Fibre: 0.5 g; Sugar 0.8 g

FRIED CHIPS

5 minutes

20 minutes

4

INGREDIENTS

- Salt
- 1 kg of potatoes, peeled, cut into 1cm batons
- Oil spray (vegetable or sunflower works best)
- Other optional seasoning
- Your favourite dip

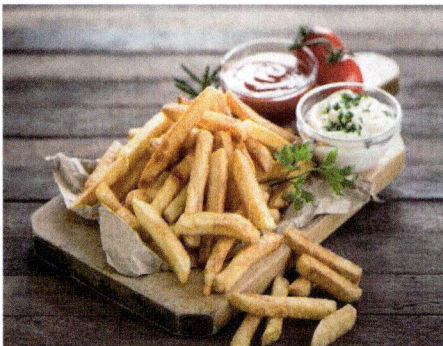

DIRECTIONS

1 Preheat to 180°C. Rinse the chips in cold water then pat them dry.
2 Place the chips into the Air Fryer basket and spray with oil. Sprinkle them with salt and any other seasoning you want, then shake the basket.
3 Air fry for 20 minutes, shake the chips halfway through to ensure even cooking. After it finishes, if the chips are not well cooked, place them back inside for 5 minutes more and continue to do so until they are good to go.
4 Serve with your favourite dip.

Nutrition: Calories: 192.5; Fat: 0 g; Protein: 5 g; Carbs: 43.5 g; Fibre: 5 g; Sugar: 2 g

COURGETTE STICKS

10 minutes   20 minutes   4

INGREDIENTS

- 2 medium courgette, sliced into 1/2cm rounds
- 2 large eggs
- 90 g panko bread crumbs
- 50 g cornmeal
- 35 g freshly grated 182
- 1 tsp. dried oregano
- 1/4 tsp. garlic powder
- Pinch chilli flakes
- Salt
- Freshly ground black pepper
- Marinara, for serving

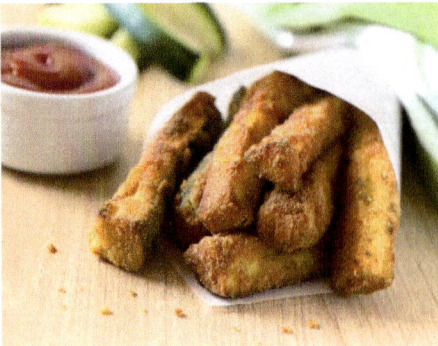

DIRECTIONS

1. Arrange the courgette on a platter lined with paper towels and pat dry.
2. Arrange the beaten eggs in a shallow bowl. Take another shallow bowl, mix cornmeal, panko, oregano, Parmesan, garlic powder, and a large pinch of chilli flakes. Add salt and pepper.
3. One at a time, dip the courgette rounds into the egg, then into the panko mixture, press to coat.
4. Arrange the courgette in an even layer, cook at 200°C 18 minutes, flip halfway through.
5. Serve warm with marinara.

Nutrition: Calories: 182; Fat: 5 g; Protein: 6.6 g; Carbs: 22 g; Fibre: 1 g; Sugar: 2 g

ONION RINGS

10 minutes

10 minutes

3

INGREDIENTS

- 2 white onions, sliced into rings
- 130 grams flour
- 2 eggs, beaten
- 130 grams breadcrumbs

DIRECTIONS

1. Cover the onion rings with flour.
2. Dip in the egg.
3. Dredge with breadcrumbs.
4. Add to the air fryer.
5. Set it to air fry.
6. Cook at 200 degs C for 10 min.

Serving Suggestions: Serve with tartar sauce.

Prep & Cooking Tips: Make ahead of time and freeze.

Air fry when ready to serve.

Nutrition: Calories 415; Fat 7 g; Carbohydrates 66 g; Protein 19 g; Fibre: 8 g; Sugar 8.5 g

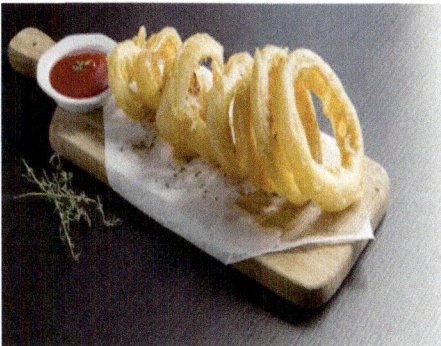

MOZZARELLA STICKS

30-60 minutes

10-30 minutes

3-4

INGREDIENTS

- 400 g block mozzarella cucina
- 2 tbsp. plain flour
- 1 tsp. garlic granules
- 1 large free-range egg
- 40g panko
- olive oil cooking spray
- salt and freshly ground black pepper

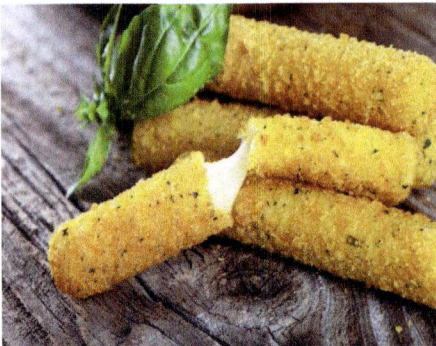

DIRECTIONS

1   Cut the mozzarella into strips, roughly 1.5 cm wide, pat dry using some kitchen paper.
2   In a shallow dish, combine flour and garlic granules. Take another dish, beat the egg and add a good amount of salt and pepper. Now spread the breadcrumbs in a third dish.
3   Roll your mozzarella strips into the flour, then into the egg, then into the flour and into the egg again, to create double coating. Check that each piece is totally covered in the flour each time. Coat well in the panko breadcrumbs.
4   Freeze 30 minutes or more, until solid.
5   Spray the bottom of your Air Fryer basket with olive oil spray, place a single layer of mozzarella sticks at the bottom. Now spray the top of the mozzarella sticks with oil, air fry 10 minutes, 200°C. Now repeat until all your mozzarella sticks are cooked, keeping each batch warm, then serve immediately.

Nutrition: Calories: 369; Fat: 23.5 g; Protein: 25 g; Carbs: 12 g; Fibre: 1 g; Sugar: 2 g

COURGETTE FRITTERS

10 minutes   10 minutes   4

INGREDIENTS

- 2 courgettes, grated
- 115 grams of Blue cheese
- 1 egg, beaten
- 1 tbsp flaxseed
- 1 tsp dried coriander
- ¼ tsp salt
- 30 grams spring onions, chopped
- 1 tsp olive oil
- 85 grams of celery stalk, diced
- 1 tbsp coconut flour

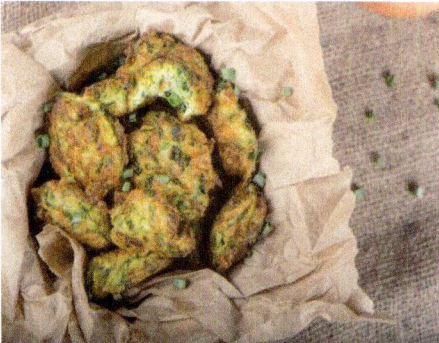

DIRECTIONS

1. Crumble Blue cheese and mix it up with grated courgettes. Add egg, flaxseed, dried coriander, salt, spring onions, diced celery stalk, and coconut flour. Then stir the ingredients with the help of the spoon until homogenous.
2. Make the fritters and sprinkle them with olive oil. After this, preheat the air fryer to 200 degs C.
3. Place the courgette fritters in the air fryer and cook them for 5 minutes. Then flip the fritters on another side and cook for 5 minutes more or until they are golden brown.

Nutrition: Calories: 164; Fat: 11.6g; Fibre: 2.8g; Carbs: 6.9g; Protein:9.6g

AUBERGINE STICKS

9 minutes   15 minutes   4

INGREDIENTS

- 1 medium aubergine
- 1 tbsp. extra-virgin olive oil
- 1 tsp. dried oregano
- 1/2 tsp. garlic powder
- Salt
- Freshly ground black pepper
- Pinch chilli flakes

DIRECTIONS

1. Take the aubergine and cut the ends off, then cut it in half (lengthwise). Now cut each half into strips about 2.5 cm thick and 7 cm long. Take a medium bowl, add oil, aubergine, and seasonings, toss to coat.
2. Arrange a single layer into the Air Fryer basket. Cook 190°C 14 minutes, until golden, shake the basket once about halfway through.

Nutrition: Calories: 58; Fat: 3.5 g; Protein: 1 g; Carbs: 6.5 g; Fibre: 3 g; Sugar: 4 g

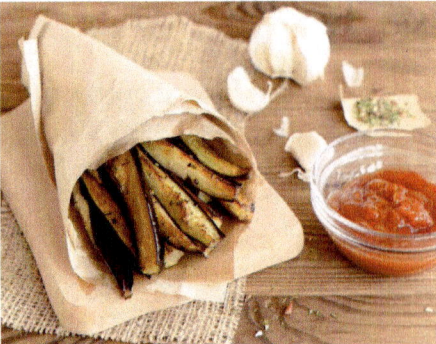

CRISPY AVOCADO CHIPS

15 minutes

10 minutes

4

INGREDIENTS

- 1 egg
- 1 tbsp lime juice
- 1/8 tsp hot sauce
- 2 tbsp flour
- 95 grams of panko breadcrumbs
- 30 grams cornmeal
- 1/4 tsp salt
- 1 large avocado, pitted, peeled, and cut into 1.2 cm slices
- Cooking Spray

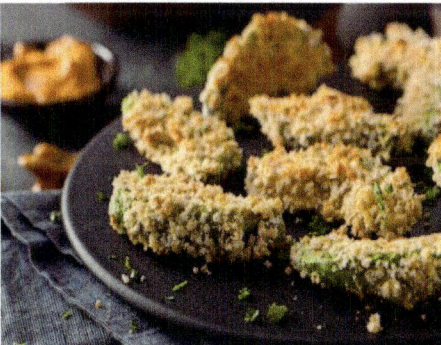

DIRECTIONS

1. Whisk together the egg, hot sauce, and lime juice in a small bowl.
2. Place now the flour on a sheet of wax paper. In a separate sheet of wax paper, combine the cornmeal, breadcrumbs, and salt.
3. Dredge the avocado slices one at a time in the flour, then in the egg mixture, finally roll them in the bread crumb mixture to coat well.
4. Place the breaded avocado slices in the air fry basket and mist them with cooking spray.
5. Place the basket on the air fry position.
6. Select Air Fry, set to 199 degs C, and set time to 10 min.
7. When cooking is complete, the slices should be nicely browned and crispy. Transfer the avocado slices to a plate and serve.

Nutrition: Calories 232; Fat 10 g; Carbohydrates 27.5 g; Protein 7 g; Fibre: 5.5 g; Sugar 3 g

ROASTED POTATOES

< 30 minutes

30-60 minutes

2

INGREDIENTS

- 2 large floury potatoes (approximately 450g)
- salt, to taste
- 1 tbsp. olive oil

DIRECTIONS

1 Peel, quarter your potatoes, then boil them in a saucepan of salted water for 15 minutes (place them when the water is already boiling).
2 Now drain the potatoes, leave them to steam dry for a minute or two.
3 Toss with olive oil and a good amount of salt.
4 Air fry 30 minutes, 200°C, toss every 10 minutes.
5 Serve.

Nutrition: Calories: 232.5; Fat: 7 g; Protein: 4.5 g; Carbs: 39 g; Fibre: 4.5 g; Sugar: 1.5 g

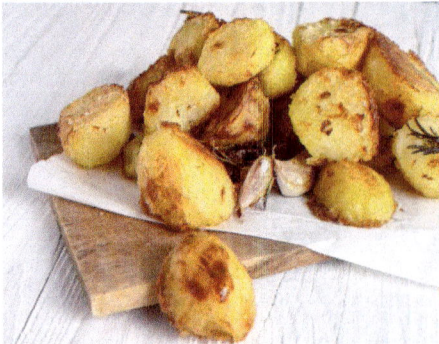

PIZZA ROLLS RECIPE

10 minutes   8 minutes   4

INGREDIENTS

- 240 g natural/Greek yoghurt
- 350 g self-raising flour
- 1 tin/carton of passata/pizza sauce (or enough to cover the dough)
- Grated cheese (Mozzarella or your favourite one)
- 1 tsp dried herbs (optional)

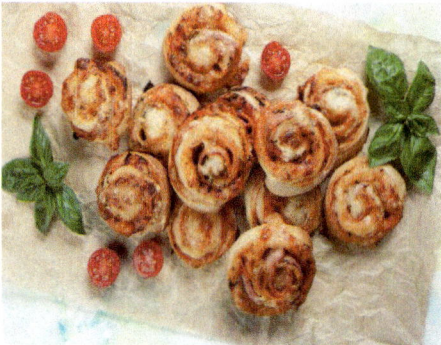

DIRECTIONS

1. Make the dough by mixing flour and yogurt in a bowl. If the mixture is too wet and sticky, add a little more flour. Add more water if it's too dry. You should be able to stretch the dough without it sticking or falling off.
2. Roll out the dough into a rectangle on a lightly floured surface. Spread the pizza sauce/passata on the dough. You can use your favourite pizza sauce or regular pasta sauce. But be careful not to make it too watery. Otherwise, it will run off the dough.
3. Sprinkle grated cheese over tomato sauce and add your favourite toppings. Carefully roll the pizza lengthwise until it forms a sausage shape. Using a sharp or serrated knife, cut pizza roll into even slices.
4. Carefully place the rolls into the air fryer basket. Air Fry at 180 °C for about 8 to12 minutes. Check halfway through to make sure it's cooking too quickly.

Nutrition: Calories: 393; Fat: 5 g; Carbohydrates: 72 g; Fibre: 3 g; Sugar: 6 g; Protein: 14 g

CRISPY PROSCIUTTO-WRAPPED ASPARAGUS

5 minutes   16 to 24 minutes   6

INGREDIENTS

- 12 asparagus spears, woody ends trimmed
- 24 pieces thinly sliced prosciutto
- Cooking Spray

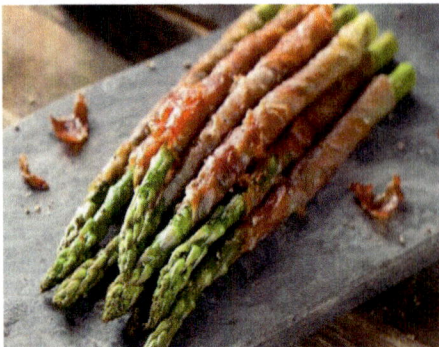

DIRECTIONS

1. Place the crisper tray on the air fry position. Select Air Fry, set the temperature to 182 degs C, and set the time to 4 min.
2. Wrap each asparagus spear with 2 slices of prosciutto, then repeat this process with the remaining asparagus and prosciutto.
3. Spray the crisper tray with cooking spray, then place 2 to 3 bundles in the crisper tray. Air fry for 4 min. Repeat this process with the remaining asparagus bundles.
4. Remove the bundles and allow to cool on a wire rack for 5 min before serving.

Nutrition: Calories 40; Fat 3 g; Carbohydrates 5g; Protein 12 g; Fibre: 3 g; Sugar 2 g

4-INGREDIENT NUTELLA BROWNIES

35 minutes   40 minutes   8

INGREDIENTS

- 150g (1 cup) plain flour
- 225g (1 cup) white sugar
- 3 eggs, lightly whisked
- 300g (1 cup) Nutella
- Cocoa powder, to dust (optional)

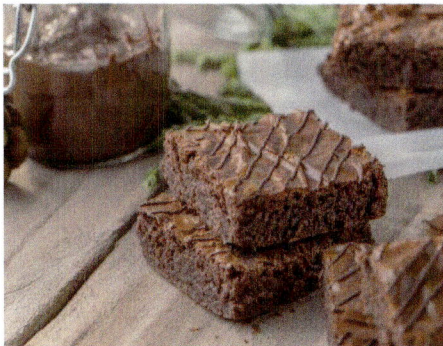

DIRECTIONS

1. Lightly grease a 20 cm round cake pan. Line the base with baking paper.
2. Whisk together the flour and sugar in a bowl with the help of a balloon whisk. Form a hole in the centre and pour the egg and Nutella into it. Using a large metal spoon, stir until everything is mixed. Transfer to the prepared baking pan and smooth the top.
3. Preheat the air fryer to 160C. Cook the brownie for about 40 minutes. To check the baking use a toothpick. Once cooked set aside and allow to cool completely.
4. Cut into pieces and serve

Nutrition: Calories: 406; Fat: 16 g; Protein: 7 g; Carbs: 58 g; Fibre: 4 g; Sugar: 38 g

LEMONY CHEESECAKE

5 minutes   25 minutes   6

INGREDIENTS

- 495 grams of ricotta cheese
- 155 grams of sugar
- 3 eggs, beaten
- 3 tbsp flour
- 1 lemon, juiced and zested
- 2 tsps vanilla extract

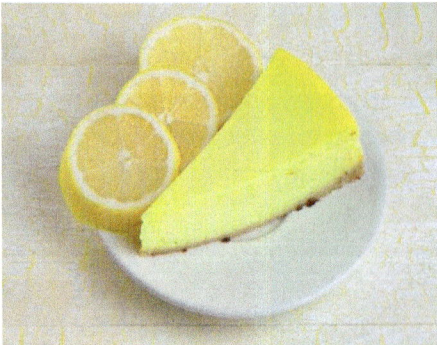

DIRECTIONS

1. In a very large mixing bowl, stir all the ingredients until the mixture reaches a creamy consistency.
2. Pour the mixture in a baking pan and place it in the air fryer grill.
3. Place the pan on the bake position.
4. Select Bake, set temperature to 160 degs C, and set time to 25 min.
5. When cooking is complete, a toothpick inserted in the center should come out clean.
6. Allow to cool for 10 min on a wire rack before serving.

Nutrition: Calories 292.5; Fat 13.3 g; Carbohydrates 29.5 g; Protein 13.3 g; Fibre: 0.4 g; Sugar 24.3 g

CLASSIC POUND CAKE

5 minutes

30 minutes

8

INGREDIENTS

- 1 stick butter, at room temperature
- 130 grams Swerve Sweetener
- 4 eggs
- 190 grams coconut flour
- 65 grams buttermilk
- 1/2 tsp baking soda
- 1/2 tsp baking powder
- 1/4 tsp salt
- 1 tsp vanilla essence
- A pinch of ground star anise
- A pinch of freshly grated nutmeg
- Cooking Spray

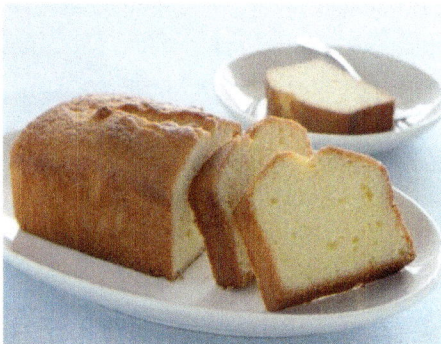

DIRECTIONS

1. Place the baking pan on the bake position. Select Bake, set the temperature to 160 degs C, and set the time to 30 min.
2. Spray the baking pan with cooking spray.
3. With an electric or hand mixer, beat butter and Swerve until creamy. One at a time, mix in the eggs and whisk until fluffy. Add now the remaining ones and stir to combine.
4. Transfer the batter to the baking pan. Bake for 30 min until the center of the cake is springy. Rotate halfway through the Cooking.
5. Let the cake to cool down in the pan for 10 min before removing and serving.

Nutrition: Calories: 155; Fat: 12 g; Fibre: 0 g; Carbs:4 g; Protein:5.6 g; Sugar: 3.6 g

CREAMY CHOCOLATE ECLAIRS

15 minutes   25 minutes   9

INGREDIENTS

Éclair Dough:
- 50 g Butter
- 100 g Plain Flour
- 3 Medium Eggs
- 150 ml Water

Cream Filling:
- 1 tsp. Vanilla Essence
- 1 tsp. Icing Sugar
- 150 ml Whipped Cream

Chocolate Topping:
- 50 g Milk chocolate (chopped into chunks)
- 1 tbsp. Whipped Cream
- 25 g Butter

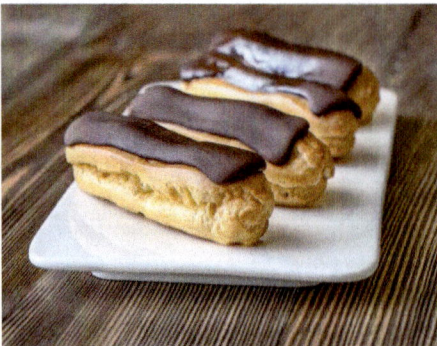

DIRECTIONS

1. Preheat the Air Fryer to 180°C.
2. While it is heating up, place the butter in the water, melt over medium heat, using a large pan, then bring to the boil.
3. Now remove it from the heat and stir in the flour.
4. Place the pan again to the heat and stir into it forms a medium ball in the middle of the pan.
5. Transfer the dough to a cold plate so that it can cool. Once it is cool beat in the eggs until you have a smooth mixture.
6. Then make into éclair shapes and place in the Air Fryer. Cook for 10 minutes on 180°C and a further 8 minutes on 160°C.
7. While the dough is cooking make your cream filling: Mix with a whisk the whipped cream, vanilla essence and icing sugar until nice and thick.
8. Leave the eclairs to cool and while they are cooling make your chocolate topping – Place the milk chocolate, whipped cream and butter into a glass bowl. Place it over a pan of hot water and mix well until you have melted chocolate.
9. Cover the tops of the eclairs with melted chocolate and then serve!

Nutrition: Calories: 181; Fat: 13 g; Protein: 4 g; Carbs: 27.5 g; Fibre: 1.5 g; Sugar: 3 g

MUFFINS WITH BLUEBERRIES

25 minutes

15 minutes

3

INGREDIENTS

- 60 grams of butter
- 60 ml of fresh whole milk
- 140 grams of flour type "00"
- 60 grams of sugar
- 1 egg
- 5 grams of baking powder
- 1/2 sachet of vanillin
- 70 grams of blueberries
- 1/4 tsp of baking soda
- 1 pinch of salt

Cooking tools:

- Baking cups for muffins

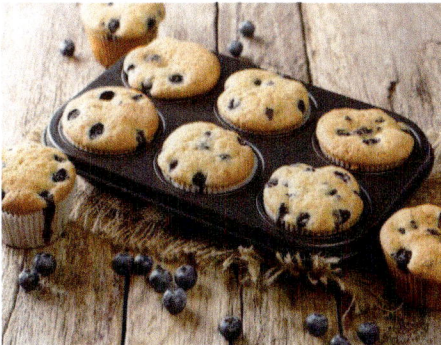

DIRECTIONS

1. Soften the butter at room temperature in the bowl. Add the sugar and then whisk vigorously until a creamy mixture is obtained.
2. Add the egg while continuing to whip.
3. Pour the milk at room temperature slowly, whipping until smooth.
4. Sift the flour into a bowl and mix it together with the baking powder, baking soda, vanillin, and salt. Add them little by little to the mixture until it is creamy and without lumps.
5. Add the blueberries to the dough.
6. Preheat the air fryer to 185 degs C.
7. Fill the baking cups with the mixture.
8. Put the cups with the dough in the basket and insert them into the air fryer.
9. Set the timer to 15 min and bake the muffins until lightly browned.

Nutrition: Calories 287; Fat 3 g; Carbohydrates 2 g; Sugar 3 g; Protein 11 g

BRITISH VICTORIA SPONGE

15 minutes   28 minutes   8

INGREDIENTS

For the Victoria Sponge:
- 100 g Plain Flour
- 100 g Butter
- 100 g Caster Sugar
- 2 Medium Eggs

For the Cake Filling:
- 2 tbsp. Strawberry Jam
- 50 g Butter
- 100 g Icing Sugar
- 1 tbsp. Whipped Cream

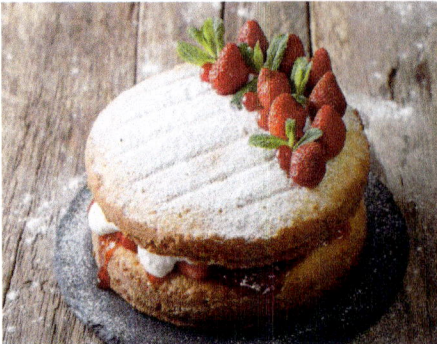

DIRECTIONS

1. Preheat the Air Fryer to 180°C.
2. Grease a baking dish.
3. Cream the sugar and the butter until light and fluffy.
4. Now beat in the eggs, add a little flour with each.
5. Now gently fold in the flour.
6. Arrange your mixture into the tin and cook for 15 minutes, 180°C, then 10 minutes, 170°C.
7. Now leave it to cool and once it is cooled slice into two equal slices of sponge.
8. Now make the filling: Cream the butter, until you have a thick creamy mixture gradually add icing sugar and whipped cream.
9. Arrange a layer of strawberry jam, then a layer of cake filling, then add your other sponge on top.
10. Serve!

Nutrition: Calories: 243; Fat: 16.5 g; Protein: 3 g; Carbs: 21 g; Fibre: 1 g; Sugar: 12 g

GOLDEN BANANAS WITH CHOCOLATE SAUCE

10 minutes

7 minutes

6

INGREDIENTS

- 35 grams corn-starch
- 35 grams plain breadcrumbs
- 1 large egg, beaten
- 3 bananas, halved crosswise
- Cooking Spray
- Chocolate sauce, for serving

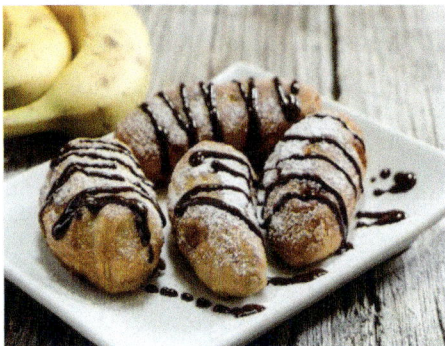

DIRECTIONS

1. Place the breadcrumbs, egg, and corn-starch in three separate bowls.
2. Roll the bananas in the corn-starch, then in the beaten egg, and finally in the bread crumbs to coat well.
3. Spritz the air fry basket with cooking spray.
4. Arrange the banana halves in the air fry basket and mist them with cooking spray.
5. Place the basket on the air fry position.
6. Select Air Fry, set temperature to 180 degs C, and set time to 7 min.
7. After about 5 min, flip the bananas and continue to air fry for another 2 min.
8. When cooking is complete, remove the bananas from the air fryer grill to a serving plate. Serve now with the chocolate sauce drizzled over the top.

Nutrition: Calories 142; Fat 1.2 g; Carbohydrates 32 g; Protein 2.5 g; Fibre: 3 g; Sugar 14 g

LEMON BISCUITS

5 minutes

5 minutes

9

INGREDIENTS

- 100 g Butter
- 100 g Caster Sugar
- 225 g Self Raising Flour
- 1 Small Lemon (rind and juice)
- 1 Small Egg
- 1 tsp. Vanilla Essence

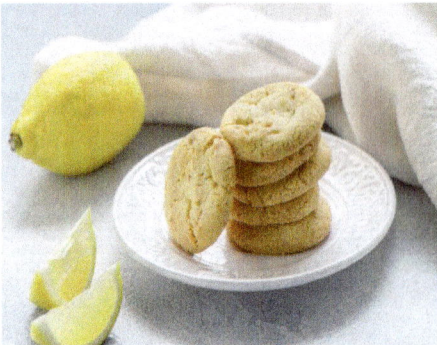

DIRECTIONS

1. Preheat the Air Fryer to 180°C.
2. Mix flour and sugar in a bowl. Add the butter and rub it in until your mix resembles breadcrumbs. Shake your bowl regularly so that the fat bits come to the top and so that you know what you have left to rub in.
3. Add the lemon rind and juice along with the egg.
4. Combine and knead until you have lovely soft dough.
5. Roll out and cut into medium sized biscuits.
6. Place the biscuits into the Air Fryer on a baking sheet and cook for five minutes at 180°C.
7. Place on a cooling tray and sprinkle with icing sugar

Nutrition: Calories: 205; Fat: 10 g; Protein: 3.5 g; Carbs: 26 g; Fibre: 2.5 g; Sugar: 10 g

SHORTBREAD CHOCOLATE BALLS

4 minutes

13 minutes

9

INGREDIENTS

- 175 g Butter
- 75 g Caster Sugar
- 250 g Plain Flour
- 1 tsp. Vanilla Essence
- 9 Chocolate chunks
- 2 tbsp. Cocoa

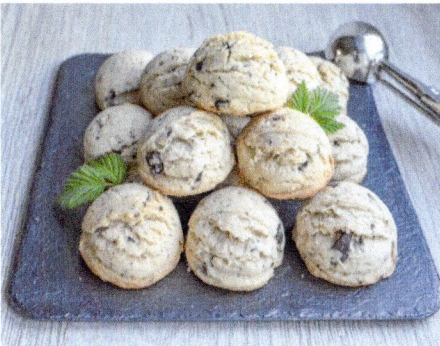

DIRECTIONS

1. Preheat your Air Fryer to 180°C.
2. Take a bowl and mix your sugar, flour, and cocoa.
3. Rub in the butter, knead well until you see a smooth dough.
4. Now divide into balls, place a chunk of chocolate into the centre of each one, make sure none of the chocolate chunk is showing.
5. Place your chocolate shortbread balls onto a baking sheet in your Air Fryer. Cook them at 180°C for 8 minutes and then a further 5 minutes on 160°C so that you can make sure they are cooked in the middle.
6. Serve!

Nutrition: Calories: 297; Fat: 18 g; Protein: 4 g; Carbs: 31 g; Fibre: 3.5 g; Sugar: 10 g

INDEX

CREDITS

Icon made by Pixel perfect from www.flaticon.com

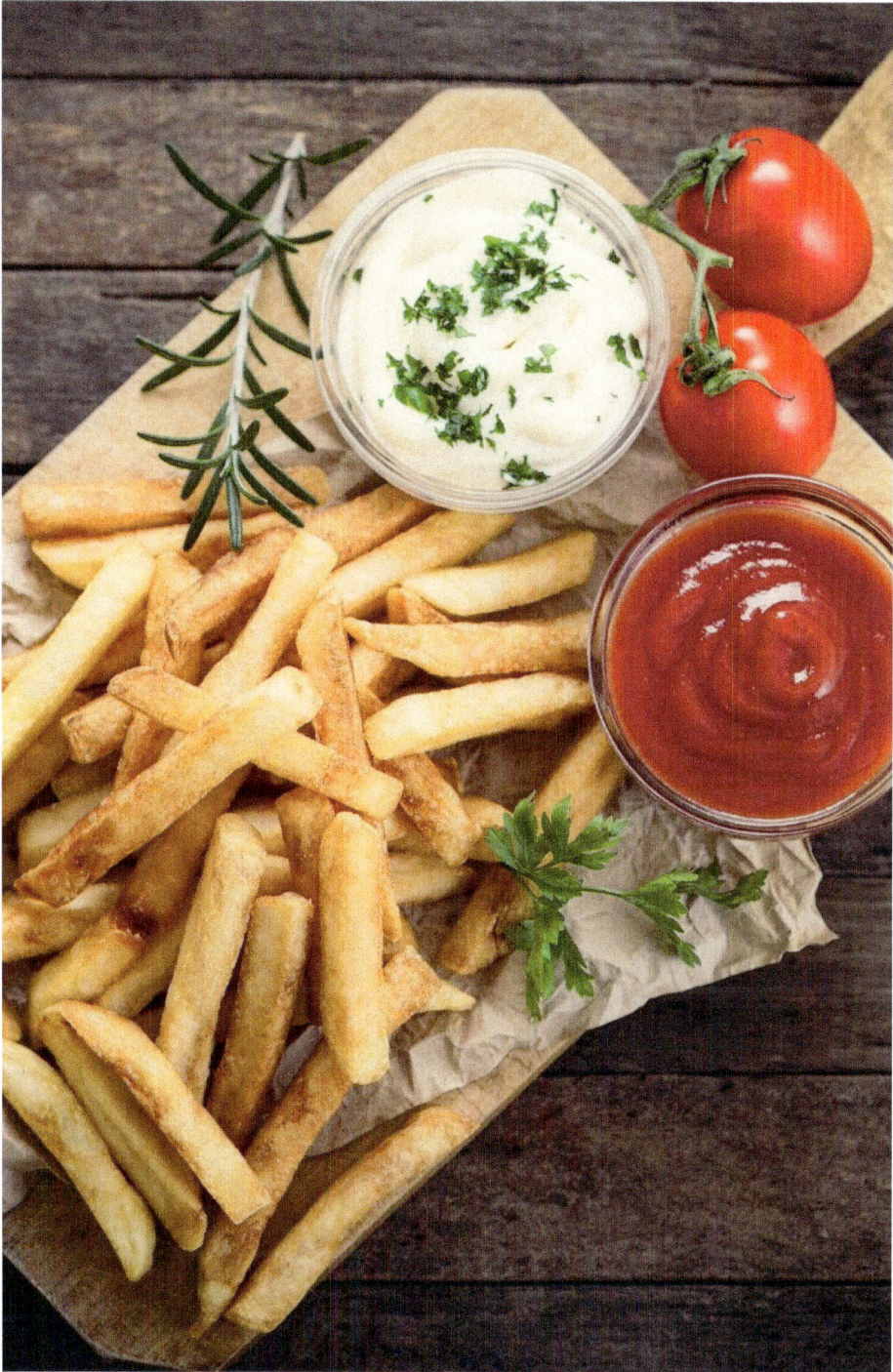

Printed in Great Britain
by Amazon